The
Natural
Healing
·ANNUAL·

1985

The Natural Healing ·ANNUAL·

1985

Edited by
Mark Bricklin
Executive Editor, PREVENTION® **Magazine**

Written by the Staff of Rodale Press

 Rodale Press, Emmaus, Pennsylvania

ISBN 0-87857-536-7   hardcover
2   4   6   8   10   9   7   5   3   1   hardcover

Contents

Protecting and Restoring Your Good Health

A New Code of Practice for Doctors
The People's Medical Society, a new nonprofit group,
is asking physicians to show their clients a little more

Prescription for Addiction
Street drugs aren't the only kind that can lead to
addiction. Today's educated consumer (or doctor)
must know that many medications have the potential

Good News Addendum

We're All Getting Younger
The old concepts of what it's like to be 40, or 50, or
75, are as outdated as the Charleston. Experts agree:

NOTICE

The information and ideas in this book are meant to supplement the care and guidance of your physician, not to replace it. The editor cautions you not to attempt diagnosis or embark upon self-treatment of serious illness without competent professional assistance. An increasing number of physicians are ready to cooperate with clients who want to improve their diet and lifestyle; if you are under professional care or taking medication, we suggest discussing this possibility with your doctor.

Introduction: Natural Healing in 1985

The knowledge of natural healing gained this year is perhaps greater than in any previous year. Yes, even in the age of high-tech, the interest scientists and doctors are evincing in drugless, knifeless healing is rising rapidly.

As you skim through this new edition of *The Natural Healing Annual,* you'll see how true that statement is. You'll read of bold, new insights such as:

- Why some fats are actually good for our hearts
- Why diet holds the promise of boosting the weak immune systems of the elderly
- Which foods seem most likely to trigger headaches in people with food allergy
- How nutrition can help prevent fibrocystic disease, and even cancer of the breasts
- How diet—and not just salt—can play a critical role in heading off high blood pressure

And of course, there's so much more—chapters and chapters of good, new, useful information

Interestingly, the doctors doing this research are, for the most part, not those who would identify themselves as "natural healers," or even "investigators of drugless therapy." No, these scientists have just as many computers, scanners, analyzers and blinking lights in their laboratories as any other high-tech scientist. It's just that they've taken a new direction. We call it natural healing. A doctor I know, who would break out in a cold sweat if that phrase were used in the same sentence as his name, puts it like this: "Many researchers are busy fashioning what we used to call 'new weapons against disease.' I guess some people still use that kind of language. I find it much more exciting to find what the body does naturally to defend and repair itself, and then figure out how to get behind those forces and *push.*"

Many doctors and the people who give doctors research grants seem to share that philosophy. Call it holistic medicine, conservative care, natural healing, or what you will—it all comes down to a belief that working *with* the body makes more sense than working *against* it.

But there's another aspect to this upsurge in natural medicine, one that's not quite so positive. It has to do with a sense that technology-intensive modern medicine has already peaked and is having a hard time just to keep from going into a tailspin.

Use of drugs, for example, plateaued some years ago. Consumers seem less anxious to take pills and doctors less eager to prescribe them. Increasing awareness of side effects and addictive potential (see "Prescription for Addiction"), as well as the failure to bring new "miracle drugs" like the antibiotics of the 50s onto the market, have been blamed (or credited, depending on your point of view).

People are spending less time in the hospital, too. The reduction isn't enormous, but many see a trend in the making. Meanwhile, a growing surplus of doctors finds itself with a population that is not exactly busting down the doors for treatment.

Despite these trends, the cost of medical care continues to spiral upward. But now people are fighting back. The government is setting strict limits on how much it pays for certain kinds of treatment. Insurance companies are encouraging second opinions before surgery. Many businesses are cutting back on free health insurance and entering into special agreements with doctors who promise to keep costs down. And all this may be just the beginning. New research has shown that surgical rates often vary dramatically from city to city, with no medical rationale whatsoever. Rather, the "practice style" of different areas seems to encourage one group of doctors to perform operations for reasons that another group of doctors would view as trivial or, at best, subjective. When these findings become known to the public, tremendous resentment may ensue. And if political leaders make an issue out of excessive surgery, we may witness the most heated debate over health policy in our history.

In this context, the *Natural Healing Annual* for 1985 becomes more than just a collection of facts and theories. It is part of the Big Answer that must be formulated in response to the question: Where is health care going?

Many of the pieces are here, right at your fingertips. The importance of good nutrition ... understanding what makes your body strong and what makes it weak ... techniques for better health that any person can use right at home ... sensible ways to keep fit ... some basic how-to's of self-care ... and a close look at how the changing medical system is affecting you, right now.

Please enjoy your new Annual!

Nutritional Healing Newsfront

Mind Rejuvenators

When asked a few years ago to name three wishes, scientist and novelist Isaac Asimov answered: to live so happily and effectively that no one would mourn his passing, to leave this world knowing that civilization would survive into the 21st century and beyond, and, finally, not to outlive his intelligence—that is, to remain productive and quick-witted to the end, without senility.

Like the 65-year-old Dr. Asimov, most of us worry about the possibility of mental decline in later life. We can tolerate the predictable aspects of the aging process—mild forgetfulness, blurred near vision, difficulty hearing—but none of us wants to be among the estimated 15 percent of those over 65 who suffer from some degree of senility.

And for the most part, there's nothing that says we must.

Doctors once accepted senility as one of the irreversible penalties of old age, but some now say the opposite: that in many cases the symptoms of senility can be prevented or reversed.

If there were a contest for the anti-senility "nutrients of the year," the annual prize might be awarded to vitamin B_6 and copper. Last year, two University of Texas nutritionists reported the remarkable news that a deficiency of B_6 or copper in young rats causes some of the same kind of brain cell abnormalities as those seen in senile humans. The results implied that those two nutrients might prevent mental decline.

1

Science, of course, is never that simple. But the evidence seems striking. The researchers found, among other things, that in rats and humans, the dendrites—delicate, branching roots that carry electrical impulses from one brain cell to another—tend to shrivel up and die when deprived of B_6 or copper. Without the all-important dendrites, brain circuitry breaks down (*American Journal of Clinical Nutrition,* April, 1983).

Though the rats were fed a diet skimpier in the two nutrients than any human diet would be, the researchers said that a mild deficiency of those nutrients over the years could have the same devastating effect. The Texas researchers, Elizabeth Root, Ph.D., and John Longenecker, Ph.D., recommended getting adequate amounts of B_6, copper and other nutrients into the diet as soon as possible for the sake of prevention. (Liver is a fine source of both.)

"If you catch these changes early, then you might prevent some of the neurological damage from occurring," Dr. Root says. "But it's not just B_6 and copper. People who have a poor diet in general are the most likely to get in trouble. We're starting some more experiments on the possible effects of deficiencies in magnesium and folate, two nutrients that also come up low in most diet surveys."

Experiments with rats are one thing, but what about studies of people like you and me? What about people who feel fairly fit mentally, but who want to be even sharper in the years ahead? What about people who want to learn how to use a home computer or write a book when they retire—or just keep their bridge game sharp? Can nutrition give them the extra edge they want?

Actually, there's recent evidence that physically healthy people over age 60 can be measurably keener of mind than their peers if they maintain sufficient dietary levels of vitamins B_{12} and C, folate and riboflavin. Even mild, virtually unnoticeable deficiencies of those nutrients can mean less-than-optimum brain function.

At the University of New Mexico, senility experts Jean M. Goodwin, M.D., and her husband, James S. Goodwin, M.D., and others placed advertisements in newspapers and on TV and radio in the Albuquerque area asking for volunteers for an experiment. Each volunteer had to be at least 60 years old, free of all serious diseases and not on medication. After a screening process, the Goodwins chose 260 men and women between the ages of 60 and 94 from various social and income levels.

All the volunteers gave a sample of their blood and filled out a three-day food diary stating exactly what they ate during that period. Taken together, the blood test and diet survey showed the researchers almost exactly what each person's levels of most vitamins and minerals were.

After this process, the volunteers underwent two mental-performance tests. In the first one, a researcher read a one-paragraph story to each person and asked him to repeat it as quickly and accurately as possible. A half hour later, the volunteers had to recite the paragraph from memory, with no cues. The second test measured each person's ability to solve nonverbal problems and to think abstractly.

The researchers fed all the test scores and nutritional profiles into a computer and waited to see if good nutrition would correlate with quicker thinking. It turned out that the volunteers with the lowest B_{12} and C levels scored worst on the memory test. Those with the lowest levels of B_{12}, C, folate and riboflavin did worst on the problem-solving test (*Journal of the American Medical Association,* June 3, 1983).

"We showed that in a population of healthy older people, those people who had a deficient intake and low blood levels of certain vitamins scored significantly worse on the tests," Dr. Jean Goodwin says. "Our recommendation is that everyone maintain an adequate intake of those nutrients."

"Giving older people extra vitamins sounds to us like a sensible course," Dr. James Goodwin adds. "Studies in nursing homes have shown that when you put half the residents on a multivitamin and the other half on a placebo [dummy pill], the staff will eventually be able to tell, with great accuracy, which half was supplemented and which wasn't. The group on the vitamins is always 'doing better.'"

One of the nursing-home studies that Dr. Goodwin refers to took place at a long-term care hospital in Leeds, England. It showed that a supplement of vitamin C could, in many cases, help even people who are weak and listless to actually improve mentally and physically.

The trial involved 115 men and women, ages 59 to 97. Half of the group received a plain soft drink every day and the other half a soft drink with 1,000 milligrams of vitamin C added to it. The experiment lasted 28 days, and the medical staff, not knowing which group was which, observed the patients to see whose appetite, interest in the life around them and general demeanor changed for better or worse.

It turned out that, in less than a month, there was greater improvement in the supplemented group. On the average, they gained more weight and became more active than usual. Some of the patients who had seemed beyond help surprised the staff with their improvements (*Lancet,* February 24, 1979).

Thiamine may also keep the brain thinking straighter and younger. An orthopedic surgeon in England thinks that thiamine deficiency can cause confusion and that confusion can lead to stumbles and broken bones.

The surgeon, M.W.J. Older, M.D., had noticed that people who came to him for hip and thighbone surgery all experienced a dip in their thiamine levels as a result of the stress of the operation. He also noticed that until the thiamine shortage passed, the patients suffered a bout of confusion.

Digging a little deeper, Dr. Older found that patients who came in for *elective* hip surgery—planned in advance, that is—weren't thiamine deficient before the operation, and their postsurgical thiamine deficiency didn't last as long. But the patients with *emergency* fractures, he discovered, were deficient before, during and after their operations. That raised the possibility that preoperative thiamine-related confusion may even have helped cause the emergencies.

"Mental confusion in the elderly awaits further study," Dr. Older notes, "but our data support the concept that thiamine deficiency may be a contributory factor to postoperative confusion. We . . . suggest that the causation of the fracture itself may be attributable to thiamine deficiency, with confusion precipitating the fall" (*Age and Aging,* 1982).

Good nutrition may even help people suffering from

Alzheimer's disease. This most-feared form of senility strikes in middle age and gradually destroys its victims mentally and physically. Alzheimer's is regarded as unexplainable and untreatable, but there is hope.

"Let's say that someone has a mild case of Alzheimer's," explains geriatric specialist Charles H. Weingarten, M.D., of McLean Hospital in Massachusetts. "They may fall into poor dietary habits that make the situation worse. You may not be able to reverse the disease. But good nutrition might enable that person to function better. It might make a significant difference in the amount of care a person requires—perhaps even allowing someone to stay at home rather than being institutionalized."

Omega-3: An Update on the New Heart Helper

Thou Shall Not Eat Shellfish, For It Hath Cholesterol. Remember this dietary commandment legislated by science?

It may have just been rescinded by something that has been changing minds and turning heads in the scientific community for over a decade—fish oil.

The news comes from William E. Connor, M.D., and a colleague at Oregon Health Sciences University in Portland. There they put a group of patients on control diets that were very low in cholesterol, then later on diets high in shellfish (and therefore high in cholesterol). To gauge the effects of the regimens, the researchers monitored the levels of cholesterol and triglycerides (circulating fats) in the patients' blood. And the results were just what shellfish lovers want to hear: Overall, the two kinds of diets had virtually the same impact on both blood factors (*Metabolism,* October, 1982).

"This means that eating moderate amounts of shellfish—3 or 4 ounces a day—is perfectly acceptable," says Dr. Connor.

To some people that makes about as much sense as a flat earth. Research has shown time and again that cholesterol-rich foods drive up cholesterol in the blood, so what's so different about shrimp and lobster and scallops?

The big difference is a class of polyunsaturated fatty acids called omega-3, says Dr. Conner. They're the healthy-heart factors found mostly in fish oils, including the oil in shellfish. Among researchers they've earned a reputation as arch foes of elements that clog the circulation.

"The implication of our findings," says Dr. Connor, "is that the omega-3 fatty acids helped neutralize the impact of the high-cholesterol shellfish diets."

And so it goes. Reports like this have been coming in for 12 years, consistently defining certain elements of fish oils as potent forces for coronary health.

First came news that Greenland Eskimos were practically immune to heart disease despite diets loaded with fat, a known cause of heart trouble. The natives ate staggering amounts of whale blubber, seal and fatty fish, but appeared to have some of the healthiest hearts in the world. Then there was word that scientists had found a clue: The Eskimos had high levels of omega-3 fatty acids in their blood—substances derived directly from their marine food. It soon became clear that the fatty acids might somehow be compensating for the fatty meals. Researchers had uncovered a dietary ally in the war on heart disease.

It wasn't long after this first bit of detective work that investigators figured out which members of the omega-3 class were chalking up most of the good deeds. Scientists called them eicosapentanoic acid (EPA) and docosahexanoic acid (DHA). In patient after patient, researchers pitted these against high levels of cholesterol and triglycerides as well as excessive blood clotting, a process that can cause a heart attack or stroke. And EPA and DHA almost always came out ahead.

Consequently, the questions surrounding omega-3 today are more intriguing than ever. Just how far can fish oil go toward prevention of heart disease? Can omega-3 do any more for your heart than other polyunsaturated fatty acids? Are omega-3 supplements just as good as a seafood diet? How much fish oil do you really need each day? Since there are now many omega-3 research projects going full tilt, the answers area getting better by the minute.

William S. Harris, Ph.D., formerly of Oregon Health Sciences University, can attest to that. He and his colleagues may have just settled a scientific argument that's been around for years—whether polyunsaturated fish oil is better for your heart than polyunsaturated vegetable oils. Researchers have known for two decades that moderate intakes of such vegetable oils could push down cholesterol levels, but can fish oil do just a good a job—or better?

To find out, Dr. Harris and his colleagues put seven people on three consecutive diets, each containing equal amounts of cholesterol and 40 percent of their calories in fat. A control diet imitated the American standard, making up its 40 percent in saturated fat. Another of the diets got its fat from polyunsaturated safflower and corn oil. And the third diet had its fat derived from salmon and salmon oil, both rich in EPA and DHA.

The researchers checked the subjects' levels of cholesterol and triglycerides at each step of the way. And when all the data were in, there was plenty to think about. The salmon and the vegetable-oil diets reduced cholesterol by about the same margin—an average of 11 percent below control-diet levels. But the salmon regimen did something that its vegetable oil counterpart couldn't: It forced down triglycerides. It reduced triglycerides an amazing 33 percent below control levels (*Metabolism*, February, 1983).

"No other polyunsaturated oils have been able to get triglyceride levels to drop in this way," says Dr. Harris. "So the impact of the fish-oil diet is really significant. For a person with high triglyceride levels, a 33 percent reduction would be an important change toward better cardiovascular health."

But there was more meaning embedded in the study than this. With the information the researchers had acquired, they were able to directly compare the effects of the two major classes of polyunsaturated fatty acids—omega-3 and omega-6 (the principal cholesterol-lowering agent in polyunsaturated vegetable oils).

"There's no question," says Dr. Harris. "Gram for gram, omega-3 fatty acids were far more potent than omega-6 fatty acids, not only in reducing triglycerides but in lowering cholesterol levels as well."

A group of scientists in Munich would no doubt salute this kind of research, for they've been scrutinizing omega-3 themselves—but from a different angle. They've been looking at the effect that this class of fatty acids has on something called platelet function, that secretive process of the blood that can tilt the scales between circulatory health and heart attack or stroke.

Platelets are those tiny blood elements so crucial to the clotting process. When you cut yourself, you need them there at the wound. Otherwise you want them to stay loose and out of mischief—to not aggregate, or clump up, choking off the flow of blood, begging for some coronary catastrophe.

But sometimes platelets become too "sticky" and start to aggregate at the wrong times. Or there's an overabundance of thromboxane in the bloodstream, a substance that sets platelets to clumping and causes vessels to constrict.

These are the problems that the West German researchers hoped omega-3 fatty acids could take on. And in perhaps the most definitive study on the subject to date, they showed that these simple derivatives of fish oil are up to the job.

For 25 days they supplemented the diets of a group of men with daily doses of nearly three tablespoons of cod-liver oil— rich in EPA and DHA. Then they ran a battery of tests to evaluate the men's cardiovascular systems, particularly the action of platelets. (For the sake of comparison, the men also took the tests either just before the 25-day trial or a month after.) And in factors measuring clotting activity, the men registered significant improvements because of their fish-oil intake. Platelet aggregation decreased, the production of thromboxane went down, the number of platelets diminished, and bleeding times even increased, another indication that risk of dangerous clotting was reduced (*Circulation,* March, 1983).

"The findings," say the investigators, "paralleled observations in native Eskimos, who have unique nutrition and low morbidity from atherothrombotic disease [heart trouble caused by fatty deposits and blood clots]."

But the biggest surprise of all was what the fish oil did for the men's blood pressure: It actually pulled it down. While they were taking the cod-liver oil, their systolic blood pressure dropped an average of nearly 10 points.

And, the researchers say, there were no side effects at all from the treatment, even though three tablespoons of cod-liver oil is normally an excessive dose, containing exceptionally large amounts of vitamins A and D.

Omega-3 fatty acids, the researchers note, may be a new preventive for atherothrombotic disease—a preventive that should be stacked against the best conventional therapies currently available, including antiplatelet drugs and omega-6 fatty acid diets.

But whose palate can possibly cozy up to the taste of cod-liver oil? And who can eat fish every day without developing an aversion to anything that swims?

Soon after fish oil started getting rave reviews from scientists around the world, people no doubt started asking such questions. And it wasn't long before somebody synthesized an answer—the fish-oil supplement, omega-3 marine concentrates.

But can the supplement do the same favors for your heart as salmon steaks or fish-liver oil? Only in the last five years have researchers been trying to figure that out. Finally there's enough solid data to shed some light on what fish-oil supplements can and cannot do.

Here's a report that reflects much of what we now know. Reginald Saynor, a leading omega-3 scientist in Sheffield, England, discloses that he's been conducting research with a fish-oil concentrate since 1980, and that he now has 150 people who've been supplementing their diets with it for up to three years. "The participants," he says, "include patients who have had myocardial infarction [heart attack], patients with angina, and symptomless volunteers. Some patients had had coronary artery bypass surgery or coronary dilatation.

"After the subjects had been taking the oil for two years,

the serum triglyceride, which fell sharply during the first few weeks, remained low and within normal limits. The total serum cholesterol was significantly lower after two years and the HDL cholesterol [the good kind] was significantly higher" (*Lancet,* June 11, 1983).

There's a limit, of course, to how much fish oil a person who is not related to seals can consume. Polyunsaturated vegetable oils, therefore, still appear to be a most valuable ally in promoting circulatory health. A big green salad tossed with oil and herb vinegar, served along with your baked or broiled fish—*that's* good eating!

Healing with Vitamin B_6

It began as just another offbeat case of side effects from medical treatment, but that's not how it turned out.

A 65-year-old woman was being treated for heart trouble with a drug (amiodarone) that causes an odd physical reaction. Doctors call the side effect photosensitivity, a malady in which even short exposure to sunlight causes itching, rashes or, in the woman's case, sunburn.

This time, however, an unusual antidote was prescribed: pyridoxine (vitamin B_6). When the woman was given daily doses of the nutrient along with her heart medication, her photosensitivity lessened.

The same thing happened with two other coronary patients who mixed B_6 and the same heart drug. And according to the medical investigator of these three cases, the B_6 "in no way impaired the desired pharmacological effects of amiodarone" (*Lancet,* January 7, 1984).

Is anyone surprised by such a finding? Certainly not researchers who know B_6 well. To them this new report will be only the latest outcrop of B_6 data in the landscape of nutritional research, an expanse already dotted with evidence of the nutrient's influence. They've seen the studies showing that B_6 may relieve asthma and hyperactivity in children, ease premenstrual tension and swelling, help prevent recurrence of bladder cancer, decrease depression in women taking birth control pills, reverse the nerve disorder called carpal tunnel syndrome and help impede the development of atherosclerosis.

In short, they know about the nutrient's versatility. Perhaps more then any other vitamin, some scientists say, B_6 is multifunctional and multifaceted.

"It's not at all astonishing that vitamin B_6 can affect so many different physical conditions that seemingly have nothing to do with one another," says Alan Gaby, M.D., Maryland physician and author of *A Doctor's Guide to Vitamin B₆* (Rodale Press, 1984). "The nutrient is a cofactor [biological activator] for at least 50 enzymes responsible for hundreds of biochemical tasks. Without B_6 the enzymes couldn't do their jobs, and body chemistry would break down in countless ways. With B_6 the biological functions can be activated and maintained."

Adults and infants, pregnant and menstruating women, body and mind—B_6's range of operations stretches far and wide. And researchers have been busy documenting it inch by inch.

And sometimes case by case. One of the more recent examples is found in a case report from doctors at Arlington Hospital in Arlington, Virginia—a scientific account that lends support to some B_6 studies done ten years ago.

Subject: schizophrenia. "An 18-year-old male entered the emergency room and was diagnosed as having acute catatonic schizophrenia," says Lawrence D'Angelo, M.D., one of the investigating doctors. "He showed signs of restlessness, insomnia, mental confusion, anorexia, hallucinations, psychomotor retardation and other symptoms. But we could find no evidence of organic brain damage, drug toxicity or any other specific cause for his condition—even after about three weeks of intensive medical investigation."

The doctors tried antipsychotic drugs on the patient, discontinued them because of severe side effects, tested the patient some more, then considered B_6. "We knew about other psychiatric case reports involving B_6," says Dr. D'Angelo. "So we started the patient on a daily B_6 regimen."

The dosage was 150 milligrams three times a day, then 500

milligrams per day—a therapeutic intake far above normal levels. The Recommended Dietary Allowance (RDA) is 1.8 to 2.2 milligrams. (*Because evidence suggests very large doses can be dangerous, you should never exceed 50 milligrams daily unless advised to do so by a knowledgeable physician.*) Within 48 hours after the dose was increased, the patient started to improve—and kept improving as long as he stayed on the nutrient therapy.

"Over a period of seven months, most of the patient's symptoms went away," Dr. D'Angelo told us. "He thought more logically and clearly and didn't demonstrate any of the abnormal behavior he had when he first came to the hospital."

But when he reduced his B_6 intake . . . relapse. He was virtually back where he started. And only the high therapeutic dose of the nutrient could bring him back toward normal.

Do the investigators understand why B_6 had such a profound effect? Not yet, but they do know that B_6's power could not be due to a single biological action. Vitamin B_6, they say, causes a whole spectrum of biochemical actions in the brain, and such multiplicity is required to affect the bundles of symptoms known as schizophrenia (*Biological Psychiatry,* vol. 18, no. 11, 1983).

No doubt it was news of B_6's brain work that prompted scientists to test the nutrient against seizures, those neural disturbances that dim consciousness and foment convulsions.

Recently at Kobe University in Japan, researchers administered high doses of B_6 to 19 children suffering from uncontrollable seizures and 17 of them improved. Three had complete relief from seizures, six showed short-term absence of seizures and eight experienced fewer seizures and improved brain waves. Overall it took only 2 to 14 days for the B_6 to have a positive impact (*Brain and Development,* vol. 5, no. 2, 1983).

Unfortunately, because of the high doses involved, some of the children had temporary side effects. But a report from David S. Bachman, M.D., of Columbus Children's Hospital in Columbus, Ohio, suggests that such high intakes may not always be necessary.

Dr. Bachman documents a case of an eight-month-old boy with a history of seizures who did not respond to standard antiseizure medication. The boy did, however, respond to something not so standard.

"He was given 50 milligrams of intravenous pyridoxine," says Dr. Bachman, "and the seizures stopped within minutes. He remained seizure-free for the next six days, when seizure activity recurred and again promptly stopped with intravenous administration of pyridoxine."

For the next 22 months the boy got 25 milligrams of oral pyridoxine daily and had no seizures at all. Then his nutrient therapy was discontinued, and the seizures began all over again. When he was put back on pyridoxine, the seizures vanished (*Annals of Neurology,* December, 1983).

"At age six," Dr. Bachman concludes, "he remains seizure-free on a daily dose of 25 milligrams of pyridoxine."

In B₆ research there's a growing number of such upbeat conclusions. Here's one that reveals a side to B₆ that most people have never seen: "This case represents another anecdotal report of the amazing result of pyridoxine therapy in the treatment of herpes gestationis."

So says Craig G. Burkhart, M.D., a dermatologist practicing in Toledo, Ohio. The problem he's referring to is a rare skin disorder that afflicts pregnant women, bringing blisters, severe itching and—no one knows why—an increase in fetal mortality. And the case in question is that of a 26-year-old expectant mother who had the blisters on her abdomen and thighs.

The usual treatment for the disease is steroid drugs like prednisone, but such therapy can be risky for mother and fetus. So this time Dr. Burkhart prescribed large daily doses of vitamin B₆—and within two weeks new blisters stopped forming and old ones receded.

The woman continued her B₆ intake right up to the birth of her healthy baby girl, then stopped—and the blisters started. She then got back on the B₆, and the herpes went into another remission (*Archives of Dermatology,* August, 1982).

In the past, a few other doctors have tested B₆ against this malady and also found it effective. The nutrient's big selling point, though, may be its relatively benign character. It's necessary to watch out for side effects from large doses of B₆, says Dr. Burkhart, but the nutrient is still much safer than steroids.

FOOD SOURCES OF
VITAMIN B₆

Food	Portion Size	Vitamin B₆ (mg.)
Banana	1 medium	0.66
Salmon	3 ounces	0.63
Mackerel, Atlantic	3 ounces	0.60
Chicken, light meat	3 ounces	0.51
Beef liver	3 ounces	0.47
Sunflower seeds	¼ cup	0.45
Halibut	3 ounces	0.39
Tuna, canned	3 ounces	0.36
Broccoli, raw	1 medium stalk	0.35
Lentils, dried	¼ cup	0.29
Brown rice, raw	¼ cup	0.28
Beef kidney	3 ounces	0.24
Brewer's yeast, debittered	1 tablespoon	0.20
Filberts	¼ cup	0.18
Buckwheat flour, dark	¼ cup	0.14

SOURCES: Adapted from
Panthothenic Acid, Vitamin B₆, and Vitamin B₁₂, Home Economics
Research Report No. 36, by Martha Louise Orr (Washington, D.C.:
Agricultural Research Service, U.S. Department of Agriculture, 1969).
Composition of Foods: Fruits and Fruit Juices, Agriculture Handbook
No. 8-9, by Consumer Nutrition Center (Washington, D.C.: U.S.
Department of Agriculture, 1982).

Vitamin E
Healing Update

It took two successful test results to prove to one hard-
boiled university researcher what his teenage daughter already
knew: Vitamin E makes wounds heal faster.

When he published his studies in a distinguished journal,
he confessed sheepishly, his daughter informed him that he
was light-years behind her camp counselor, who broke open
vitamin E capsules to treat campers' cuts and scrapes. "It had

been known by all sorts of popular nutritionists," he said, "but I did not believe them."

And who could blame him? Vitamin E has been promoted as nothing short of a magical potion that restores everything from sexual potency to youth. Its widespread use led one wag at the *Harvard Medical School Health Letter* to suggest that vitamin E be classified as a "recreational drug."

All this unfortunate ballyhoo has nearly obscured the facts about vitamin E, which in this case are proving to be far more remarkable than fiction. Right now, E is being tested not only as a potential wound healer but also as an anticancer agent and as a biochemical, not magical, antidote to aging. And there is evidence that it may do all of those things because of its ability to protect healthy cells from damage.

In wound healing, scientists believe that vitamin E protects the lymphocytes, cells that produce antibodies against disease-causing organisms.

In cancer, some scientists believe E may diligently defend cell membranes against the assault of cancer-causing substances, notably the free radicals, highly unstable molecules that can scramble the genetic information the cells contain.

Those damaged cells can become, literally, an accident looking for a place to happen, starting a chain reaction that can lead to cancer.

Free radicals may play a role in aging, too. One theory— highly controversial—says that aging is not simply the inevitable ticking away of a programmed biological clock but the result of a lifetime of avoidable damage caused by these molecules running amuck.

"What E probably does is maintain the integrity of individual cell membranes," says James R. Litton Jr., Ph.D., assistant professor of biology at St. Mary's College, Notre Dame, Indiana. "If we relate aging to the degradation of cell membranes, then, the theory is, if we maintain their integrity, we live longer."

Today, that theory is still only a few steps short of fanciful. Research is limited to animals and, in Dr. Litton's case, very small animals called rotifers.

The rotifer is a tiny aquatic creature that has a head that

seems to spin like an outboard motor and a peculiar appetite for vitamin E. When the vitamin is added to a watery colony of rotifers, more of them live longer. "We never increase their longevity," Dr. Litton stresses. "But we allow more of them to live a full life, which in the case of rotifers is 20-some days. They also have more offspring. Of course, if you live longer, chances are you produce more."

The rotifer is a minute, often microscopic invertebrate that has just a little more in common with man than bacteria have. Is it possible that its reaction to vitamin E could have any human implications? "I'd be very hesitant to say that," says Dr. Litton. "But I would like to hope so."

One area of research in which the human implications have extended beyond mere hope is in vitamin E's effect on cancer. A synthetic version of the vitamin is being used with cancer patients who have failed to respond to other therapies. Researchers report "some antitumor and analgesic effects." Though hardly a major breakthrough, they admit, "even a partial response by the infusion of vitamin E alone can be considered encouraging" (*Proceedings of the Society for Experimental Biology and Medicine,* November, 1983).

The effects of E on one particular kind of cancer—breast cancer—are particularly encouraging, although the studies are limited to animals. In fact, even when E has no effect on other cancers, as in a recent British study on rats, it still lowers the incidence of breast tumors (*International Journal for Vitamin and Nutrition Research,* vol. 53, no. 3).

The connection may be dietary fat. Some epidemiological studies show a correlation between breast cancer and high fat intake. One of the end results of fat breakdown is the cell-damaging free radicals so strongly implicated in cancer. And, as we've noted, many scientists believe that vitamin E can protect the cells from free radical assault.

But the fact is, scientists don't really know why E has an effect on breast cancer. Theoretically, it could be E's stimulatory effect on the immune system—protecting the disease-fighting cells so they can do their work.

That possibility was considered by Clement Ip, Ph.D., a researcher in the department of breast surgery and the breast cancer research unit of Roswell Park Memorial Institute in Buffalo, New York. Dr. Ip used vitamin E as part of a one-two punch, along with the trace mineral selenium, on breast tumors in rats.

Vitamin E and selenium are both antioxidants, substances that protect cells from the damage caused during fat breakdown. Both have been shown in laboratory experiments to halt tumor growth.

In Dr. Ip's studies involving rats fed a high-fat diet, the vitamin E alone had no effect on chemically induced breast tumors. But when he paired vitamin E with selenium, there was a lower incidence of cancer.

Why? So little is known about vitamin E and selenium, Dr. Ip says he's not sure. But he has two theories. One is that the vitamin E, a more powerful antioxidant than selenium, protected the cells from damage caused during the breakdown of fats and created a more favorable climate for selenium to inhibit tumor growth "via some other mechanism" as yet unknown.

Dr. Ip's second theory is that vitamin E and selenium stimulated the immune system, allowing the body's own disease-battling cells to rid it of the cancer. In at least one experimental model, a deficiency of antioxidants stimulates tumor growth. More important, when vitamin E and selenium are added to the diet in quantities in excess of the recommended daily requirement, the immune system seems to be stimulated. (Caution: Very high amounts of selenium are toxic.)

Vitamin E's stimulatory effect on the immune system may have been responsible for the remarkable recovery rate of laboratory rats from both gum wounds and oral cancer in tests by researcher Gerald Shklar, D.D.S., of the department of oral medicine and oral pathology of the Harvard School of Dental Medicine in Boston.

In the gum-wound study, the rats given daily doses of vitamin E began to heal within two days of their injury. The results of the cancer study were even more astounding. "There," says Dr. Shklar, "vitamin E very significantly delayed oral cancer formation and in some cases even prevented it."

Dr. Shklar is so encouraged by his results he says he can forsee "eventually" undertaking similar studies on human subjects.

B$_{12}$—A New Nutritional Brainstorm

The patient's behavior changed quite suddenly and became increasingly bizarre. He was irritable and agitated. He was hardly sleeping at all and was hyperactive. And he had delusions that he was of great importance. In fact, he was convinced that his hometown was planning a day of celebration in his honor, and that several Hollywood celebrities would attend. When he was finally admitted to a hospital, it took six men to restrain him. And the patient was 81 years old!

His doctor performed all of the proper physical and neurological tests, but the results were normal. And all of his blood tests were normal, too. Except for one. The test for vitamin B$_{12}$ showed that he had an abnormally low level of the vitamin in his blood.

The doctor prescribed daily B$_{12}$ intravenously, and by the end of one week, the patient's mental status returned to normal. He continued to receive weekly B$_{12}$ by injection and six months later was still completely normal.

"That particular syndrome, called mania, has never before been traced to B$_{12}$ deficiency, so most general physicians may not be aware of that possibility," says Frederick Goggans, M.D., the doctor who treated that patient. "But what makes the case even more unusual is that the patient's mental problems appeared before any other signs of B$_{12}$ deficiency."

Usually, a B$_{12}$ deficiency is easy to spot, because even though it's needed in only tiny amounts (the Recommended Dietary Allowance, or RDA, is 3 *micro*grams), B$_{12}$ works for us in a big way. It's needed for the production of healthy red blood cells and for proper functioning of the nervous system.

When there's not enough B$_{12}$ to go around, the nerves and spinal cord are affected, leading to numbness and tingling in the hands and feet, and an unsteady gait. The red blood cells become enlarged and misshapen, and are unable to carry oxygen properly, which is their main job. The condition is called pernicious anemia, and other symptoms are pallor, weakness, fatigue and diarrhea. Mental problems can eventually occur, but not until much later. Or that's what doctors used to think. New reports are proving that's not always true.

At the University of North Carolina, doctors recently described the cases of two patients with psychoses (severe mental disorders) caused by vitamin B_{12} deficiencies. Both of the patients had no other symptoms of B_{12} deficiency, and both returned to normal after receiving B_{12} injections.

The doctors warn that "psychiatric manifestations may be the first symptoms of vitamin B_{12} deficiency," and they recommend that all patients with psychoses caused by brain-tissue dysfunction be checked for B_{12} deficiency (*American Journal of Psychiatry*, February, 1983).

"Even though most doctors are aware that B_{12} deficiency can lead to psychiatric symptoms, they may not be aware that it can happen before any signs of anemia," says Lorrin Koran, M.D., associate professor of psychiatry at Stanford University Medical Center.

"So upon finding normal red blood cells, a doctor may be likely to dismiss the possibility of B_{12} deficiency prematurely," adds Dr. Goggans.

How does a doctor know when to check further? "Severe mental disorders usually begin when people are in their twenties," explains Dr. Goggans, who is director of the neuropsychiatric evaluation unit at the Psychiatric Institute of Fort Worth. "So when an older person comes into the hospital with mental problems and has no prior history of a mental disorder, I'm sure to screen for B_{12} deficiency."

Other more common psychiatric problems can be caused by B_{12} deficiency, too. "Depression and dementia in the elderly are the two syndromes most classically associated with B_{12} deficiency," Dr. Goggans told us. "Dementia closely resembles senility, with its loss of intellectual function. But when it's caused by B_{12} deficiency, it's reversible." Unfortunately, many elderly people may be written off as senile when their condition is actually treatable.

"Biochemical depression is also very common in the elderly," adds Dr. Goggans. "It causes sleep and appetite disturbances, lack of energy and intellectual decline. But it's also easily treatable by standard antidepressants and is exceptionally responsive to B_{12} replacement therapy."

"We're careful to check for B_{12} deficiency in older people," says Todd Estroff, M.D., assistant director of neuropsychiatric evaluation at Fair Oaks Hospital in Summit, New Jersey. "They're especially susceptible because they don't eat well. The older person with poor teeth who tries to survive on tea and toast is more likely to develop a deficiency."

One study of 49 patients in the geriatric psychiatry unit of a Massachusetts hospital found more B_{12} deficiency than any other undiagnosed medical problem. "None of these patients had frank pernicious anemia ... nor was there evidence of peripheral neuropathy [nerve damage]," say the researchers (*Journal of the American Geriatrics Society,* December, 1982).

In another study, published by three doctors from Denmark, low values of B_{12} were found in one out of every three patients admitted to a geriatric center (*Acta Medica Scandinavica,* vol. 200, no. 4).

But the elderly aren't the only ones at risk. "I've seen teenagers with B_{12} levels so low you wonder how they can be walking," says Charles Tkacz, M.D., medical director of the North Nassau Mental Health Center in Manhasset, New York. "It's amazing they didn't need to be carried in on a stretcher. They're getting into trouble because of a junk-food/fast-food diet."

Of all foods, beef liver packs the biggest B_{12} wallop, but it's also found in other meats, fish, dairy products and eggs. Because B_{12} is found almost exclusively in foods of animal origin, anyone who avoids those foods runs the risk of developing a deficiency. That's why vegans, strict vegetarians who eat no eggs or dairy products, can become deficient if they're not careful.

But even those of us who aren't vegetarians should make extra sure to get enough B_{12}. A government study released last year showed that the amount of B_{12} we're eating has decreased dramatically over the last two decades. According to the researchers, our intake of B_{12} dropped by 8 percent during that period, more than for any other vitamin. The reason? A lower consumption of liver and dairy products, say the researchers.

The trouble is, even if you *do* eat plenty of B_{12}-rich foods, you may still end up with a deficiency. Some people can't absorb B_{12} from their digestive system because they lack what is known as *intrinsic factor,* a molecule that latches onto B_{12} and escorts it to the site on the intestinal wall where it is absorbed. Because intrinsic factor is produced in the stomach, people who have had stomach surgery are also likely candidates for B_{12} deficiency. They remain healthy only as long as they receive B_{12} injections, which bypass the digestive problems.

Other factors can upset the precarious balance of this vitally important substance, too. Cholesterol-lowering medications, potassium-replacement agents and anticonvulsants can all interfere with B_{12} absorption. And studies have shown that antiulcer drugs can have the same effect, because they reduce stomach acidity, which is important for B_{12} absorption.

"Certain parasites, such as some tapeworms, can also steal B_{12}," Dr. Koran told us.

"Luckily, vitamin B_{12} deficiency is usually among the easiest deficiencies to correct," says Dr. Tkacz. "And since depression is so common, we check everyone who is admitted to our hospital."

"My chief job is to screen patients for underlying medical illness, so everyone in my hospital gets checked for B_{12} deficiency," says Dr. Estroff. "They must get by me before they can be called psychiatric patients."

Unfortunately, if you go to your family doctor because of a mental problem, he probably won't check for B_{12}. "When most doctors see behavioral symptoms, they refer the patient to a psychiatrist," Dr. Estroff told us. "They tend not to look for physical disorders. And most psychiatrists don't look for B_{12} deficiency because they rely on the general practitioners to clear the patients medically. The way it ends up, nobody covers it.

"The result is that the patient may not receive the proper treatment," he continues. "They may be given shock treatments, antidepressants or other medication because their problems are mistakenly labeled as psychiatric."

Dr. Tkacz has found the same thing. "Some doctors don't check for vitamin deficiencies in psychiatric patients. I've seen patients who've been to four or five other doctors or hospitals before coming to our center, and it's not unusual for us to find that they have B_{12} deficiencies."

"And if you don't look for it," says Dr. Estroff, "you don't find it."

The problem is, even if the doctor does check for B_{12} deficiency, the test results may not be accurate. Several studies have shown that the usual test for B_{12}, called the radiodilution assay, is unreliable.

"The standard test measures B_{12} as well as some similar but inactive forms," Dr. Estroff explains. "So the test may show a normal result when the patient is actually deficient. That fact is not widely known by physicians and psychiatrists. There is another, more reliable test, but it's more difficult to do, takes longer and is more expensive, so most labs don't use it."

How many people may be suffering needlessly because of undiagnosed B_{12} deficiency? Dr. Koran is conducting a study that may give us some idea. "We're checking for previously undiagnosed medical illness in patients using mental health services in four California counties," he told us. "Participants in the study have a careful medical history taken and receive a complete physical examination with lab tests, including a test for B_{12}. The results of that study may give us a hint as to the extent of the problem."

"Psychiatric symptoms *can* be caused by medical illness," Dr. Estroff maintains. "B_{12} deficiency is one cause, but it's just the tip of the iceberg. It's a small aspect of a highly neglected area of medicine and psychiatry."

Why Doctors Are Excited about Carnitine

It was discovered as far back as 1905, has been scrutinized in 2,000 scientific studies and is used successfully to treat seriously ill patients of all ages. Yet most people haven't even heard of it.

Carnitine, a proteinlike nutrient manufactured in the body and available in foods, may be the best-kept secret of nutritional science.

It may also turn out to be one of the most promising, say some researchers. Indeed, some of carnitine's clinical reports sound almost too good to be true:

- After 18 years of gradual muscle disintegration, a 23-year-old woman was a quadriplegic. But daily doses of carnitine turned this slow decline around in ten days. And after eight months of carnitine treatment, her muscles were back to normal.

- A nine-year-old girl was dying of a congenital heart disorder that had already killed her three siblings. But when she was given oral carnitine, she quickly got better. After six months of daily carnitine supplements, she was reported in good health.

- A 20-year-old woman suffered from muscle weakness and deteriorated brain function. But with daily carnitine intake, she recovered completely in two months.

Such cases, however, are merely the most dramatic side of a complex substance that investigators are just now beginning to understand. Researchers have identified two types of carnitine-deficiency disease, 15 disorders accompanied by carnitine depletion and at least a half dozen ailments that may respond to carnitine supplements—including heart disease and a form of Reye's syndrome. But the medical world is still quietly mulling over the evidence, and most of it is incomplete.

"Carnitine's potential, though, now seems tremendous," says Stephen DeFelice, M.D., a New Jersey physician and pioneer in carnitine investigations. "After years of scientific apathy, carnitine research is booming."

And most of the boom owes a historical debt to a single carnitine breakthrough: the discovery that the nutrient's main function is to help the body burn fat. "Carnitine is known technically as a quaternary amine," says Dr. DeFelice. "And its most important role is to shuttle fatty acids—crucial fuel for the body—into each cell, where they can be burned for energy."

One researcher has even called carnitine a biochemical carburetor, a mechanism for regulating the amount of fuel that gets burned in the cellular engines.

All of which has inevitably led to speculation—but little evidence—that carnitine is the pill that dieters have been dreaming of. But insight into the "carburetor" function has also shed light on an array of puzzling and often fatal disorders of carnitine deficiency.

"The two categories of carnitine-deficiency disease are called systemic and myopathic," says Austin Shug, Ph.D., carnitine researcher and professor of neurology at the University of Wisconsin Medical School in Madison. "In the systemic type there's a lack of carnitine throughout the body—in blood, organs and muscles. In the myopathic type, there's adequate carnitine in the blood but not in the organs and muscles. And though the symptoms of deficiency syndromes can vary considerably—from low blood sugar to coma—both types generally involve muscle weakness and buildup of fats in the muscle fibers."

Which makes perfect sense, considering carnitine's metabolic talents. Without carnitine, energy-production centers that burn fat, like those in muscle, are disabled or shut down. Such a biological energy crisis, say researchers, would explain weakness in muscles and fat accumulation in muscle tissue.

"These carnitine-depletion diseases are more common than people might suppose," Dr. Shug told us. "They're especially prevalent among children. My colleagues and I have tested several thousand children and detected carnitine deficiencies in about 100 of them. Doctors treated most of them with carnitine and saved many lives."

Perhaps just as startling is the recent discovery that these deficiency disorders actually include a form of Reye's syndrome, the often lethal childhood disease of brain degeneration.

"Reye's, of course, is not necessarily a carnitine depletion," says Dr. Shug, "but one type of the syndrome is indeed a systemic carnitine deficiency. And Reye's children do respond to carnitine treatment."

And so do heart patients.

For years researchers had suspected that carnitine played

a crucial role in coronary health. After all, fat is the favored fuel of the heart (unlike skeletal muscles, for example, which burn both fat and carbohydrates). In the heart—one of the organs with the highest concentrations—carnitine is the stoker that shovels fat into the heart's metabolic burners. The first evidence of carnitine's friendship with the heart showed up in animal studies. They indicated that carnitine could help protect against arrhythmia (irregular heartbeat) and heart failure, and enhance normal coronary functioning. But the human studies have been even more impressive. Investigators confirmed the antiarrhythmia action and found that carnitine could also reduce angina attacks, lower triglycerides (blood fats) and raise HDL cholesterol (the beneficial kind).

Dr. DeFelice and his colleagues were among the first to use carnitine against episodes of angina. "I theorized that because carnitine could increase the fuel supply to the heart, the nutrient could normalize coronary function during an angina attack," he says. "We helped confirm this when we tested heart patients while they exercised on a treadmill. Without supplemental carnitine, their activity soon led to chest pains. But after carnitine injections, their hearts could expend more energy before angina occurred."

Researchers from the William S. Middleton Memorial Veterans Hospital in Madison, Wisconsin, found that carnitine has an even more profound effect on people with heart disease. They selected 18 patients with either angina or ischemia (blockage of blood vessels), then examined their treadmill performance after injections of carnitine or a placebo (inactive fluid). The data revealed that when the patients received carnitine, they exercised with less strain on the heart, maintained a lower heart rate and worked out longer before having chest pains (*Current Therapeutic Research*, November, 1981).

So if carnitine can protect the heart, energize the muscles and stoke the biochemical fires, shouldn't it also boost athletic performance?

"Theoretically, it should be possible," Dr. Shug says, and other investigators agree. Studies have already shown that carnitine supplements can increase the stamina and endurance of laboratory animals. And there's some evidence that hints at—but does not prove—a similar effect in humans.

But athletic considerations aside, do you under normal circumstances need to add carnitine to your diet?

Probably not, say most researchers. "Your body synthesizes a lot of its own carnitine," says Dr. DeFelice. "Plus, there's some carnitine in the foods you consume, especially meat. And there's just no hard evidence yet that a healthy person needs more carnitine than synthesis or a normal diet can provide."

Nevertheless, the available data have encouraged some (including a few carnitine researchers) to start using carnitine supplements. And thus the issue of safety has arisen.

Scientists distinguish between two forms of the nutrient and point out that one (L-carnitine) has been shown to be reasonably safe while the other (D-carnitine) may not be so benign. A recent Food and Drug Administration review of carnitine research indicates that a mixture of the two forms, called D,L-carnitine, has caused nerve and muscle problems in dialysis patients at doses of 900 to 1,200 milligrams per day. Patients not on dialysis, however, have shown no such reactions to similar doses.

These findings underscore what researchers have said all along: There's still much to learn about carnitine's impact on human physiology.

"Carnitine has value in life-threatening and serious diseases," says Dr. DeFelice. "But large doses should be taken only under a doctor's supervision."

Meanwhile, this nutrient—once mislabeled a B vitamin and relegated to nutritional obscurity—will keep scientists working overtime to see if it really is too good to be true.

Vitamin C: How Much Is Too Much?

If you listen to recent stories in the general press, there's almost *no* safe dosage level of vitamin C. And for people with certain health profiles, side effects *can* occur. Yet, according to two expert nutritional sources with whom we consulted, the benefits of vitamin C supplementation still far outweigh the possible risks of side effects.

Myriad studies have demonstrated vitamin C's protective effect against a wide variety of diseases, viruses, bacteria and toxins. It's also well known for its role in helping people recover from illness and other stresses.

But what about possible side effects? Here's a listing of the most frequently cited "risks," with an assessment of them by nutritional experts:

Calcium-Oxalate Kidney Stones • There is a possible risk of forming kidney stones, especially if you have a family history of kidney stones, according to Jonathan V. Wright, M.D., an expert on nutritional therapy from Kent, Washington. You may want to ask your doctor to test you to see if high doses of vitamin C (more than three or four grams) greatly increase your oxalate excretion. (Excess oxalate excretion may cause kidney stones.) If a problem is discovered, you can discontinue the amount of vitamin C causing it or begin taking vitamin B_6 and magnesium, which can greatly reduce oxalate stone formation from any cause, explains Dr. Wright in his book *Dr. Wright's Guide to Healing with Nutrition* (Rodale Press, 1984).

Rebound Scurvy • Some critics of vitamin C have warned that children born to mothers taking high doses can suffer from rebound scurvy, a vitamin C-deficiency disease. Also, it's been said that people who take high doses and then stop suddenly may suffer from rebound scurvy because their bodies have grown accustomed to large amounts.

However, Dr. Wright says mothers who breastfeed should not have this problem with their infants, since vitamin C is transferred through breast milk. Children who have been weaned can be given a small amount of supplemental C. Check with a nutrition-oriented doctor for the amount your child should be given.

An adult who decides to stop taking vitamin C should taper down gradually to prevent rebound scurvy, says Dr. Wright.

Red Blood Cell Breakdown • This is a rare condition, and those who are vulnerable to it have a deficiency of the enzyme G-6-PD. The deficiency is found mostly in black males and to some degree among Sephardic Jews, persons of Mediterranean descent, South American Indians, Chinese, Thais and Melanesians, according to Dr. Wright. (A blood test can detect G-6-PD deficiency.) If given extremely high doses of vitamin C *intravenously* (oral doses don't cause the same effect), such vulnerable persons can be at risk for red blood cell breakdown. However, there have been only three reported cases of this serious side effect.

Interference with Anticoagulants • If you're currently taking anticoagulant, or blood-thinning, medication, you should discuss your vitamin C supplementation with your doctor. Large doses of vitamin C can interfere with an anticoagulant's effectiveness, says Dr. Wright. You can opt to take a larger dose of the anticoagulant if you want to continue taking vitamin C.

Interference with Diagnostic Tests • Some evidence suggests that vitamin C can inhibit detection of hidden blood in the stool and urine. If you're going to have such tests, simply stop vitamin C supplementation 72 hours before the tests, advise nutrition experts Emanuel Cheraskin, M.D., D.M.D., W. Marshall Ringsdorf, D.M.D., and Emily Sisley, Ph.D., in *The Vitamin C Connection* (Harper & Row, 1983).

Diarrhea • Many experts have established a connection between high vitamin C supplementation (from three to ten grams) and diarrhea. Some doctors suggest, though, that your digestive system will gradually adapt to a high dose, according to the authors of *The Vitamin C Connection*. Otherwise, you can cut back your dosage.

The Recommended Dietary Allowance (RDA) for vitamin C is 60 milligrams. Noted vitamin authority Roger Williams recommends 250 milligrams a day if you want to play it safe. However, to help you protect against an illness that vitamin C has been shown to affect or to help you cope with one, well-known vitamin C specialists have recommended from 600 to 10,000 milligrams (ten grams) a day. Other authorities suggest that your individual health profile should be the deciding factor (e.g., if you smoke, drink, are under a lot of stress, take a lot of medication or live in a highly polluted area like Los Angeles or New York City, you probably have greater vitamin C needs than others). A nutrition-oriented doctor can help you decide what's best for you.

It's our feeling that it's best to stay below about 500 milligrams a day, except perhaps for short periods of time when somewhat more may be appropriate.

Over 40?
It's Calcium Time!

The milk mineral, the builder of bones, the maker of molars, is fast losing its ho-hum image bred in high school health classes of yesteryear.

For example: A panel of experts recently decided to rethink women's Recommended Dietary Allowance (RDA) for calcium as set by the National Research Council. The panelists, deliberating for the National Institutes of Health, proposed that the current RDA of 800 milligrams per day be bumped to a daily 1,000 milligrams before menopause and 1,500 milligrams after menopause.

Why all the fuss about more calcium for women? Osteoporosis. It's the bone-thinning, bone-fracturing disease that some experts say is virtually epidemic among older American women. For years medical people have suspected that calcium could prevent or impede the malady, and now the case for calcium therapy seems stronger than ever.

"It is by no means certain that lack of calcium causes osteoporosis," says Robert P. Heaney, M.D., expert in bone physiology at Creighton University in Omaha. "But available evidence suggests that dietary calcium may have a positive effect on the disease, which is essentially a gradual loss of bone mass. We now know that bone loss happens to everyone after age 35 or 45, but it's greatly accelerated in women past menopause. Osteoporosis is frequently the result, and calcium may counteract it."

So say several studies, including the latest one from Australia. There researchers selected 14 postmenopausal women with osteoporosis, gave them 1,000 milligrams of calcium daily for eight days, then measured the impact of the supplements on bone resorption, or degeneration. The effect was dramatic— the women showed "significant reduction in bone resorption" (*American Journal of Clinical Nutrition,* June, 1984).

Such data may be slowly changing the way doctors treat their osteoporotic patients. Most physicians now view calcium intake as an adjunct to estrogen therapy, a standard treatment for the disease. And some suggest trying calcium before resorting to estrogen, an agent whose long-term use is linked to increased risk of uterine cancer.

"Certainly the case for calcium as osteoporosis therapy isn't yet proved," Dr. Heaney admits. "But I think it's best to take the course of least risk. If we say that increased calcium is ineffective, the damage can be great if we're wrong. If we recommend increased calcium and it does nothing, no one is harmed."

But what of the case for calcium as a treatment for hypertension, the biological accomplice in thousands of American deaths? A decade has come and gone since researchers first suggested that calcium in drinking water was related to lower blood presure. And over the years the calcium/hypertension link has grown stronger in surprising ways.

One of the latest and biggest studies of the connection comes from a group of researchers at Oregon Health Sciences University in Portland and Temple University in Philadelphia. They borrowed data from a massive government study of the American population (the Health and Nutrition Examination Survey) and analyzed the information for correlations between nutrient intake and high blood pressure. In over 10,000 men and women claiming they never had hypertension, the investigators assessed blood pressure and consumption of 17 nutrients, including vitamins A and C, iron, potassium and calcium.

As it turned out, about 9 percent of the people had

hypertension, which was more consistently associated with low calcium intakes than with deficits of any other nutrient. In fact, say the researchers, "none of the hypertensive subgroups had a mean intake of calcium equal to the current recommendation" of 800 milligrams per day.

And, not surprisingly, consumption of dairy products—rich sources of calcium and potassium—was a strong indicator of whether somone over age 34 had high blood pressure. "The greater an individual's consumption of dairy products," say the investigators, "the less likely it was that he or she was hypertensive" (*Science,* June 29, 1984).

But an even more intriguing look at calcium's influence on errant blood pressure comes from a team of researchers at Cornell University Medical School in New York City. In one of the first studies to actually test the power of calcium supplements against hypertension in humans, the researchers gave 26 mildly hypertensive patients 2,000 milligrams of oral calcium for six months. The result was a "modest but consistent" drop in pressure—from an average of 161/94 at the start of the study to 154/89 six months later.

For some of the subjects, the change was even more dramatic. "The patients who started with lower levels of calcium in their blood showed the greatest decrease in pressures," says Lawrence M. Resnick, M.D., head of the research team. "In some cases, diastolic pressures dropped 10 to 20 percent. Patients with higher calcium levels, however, weren't helped at all by the calcium supplements. So the nutrient can benefit some, but not all, hypertensives."

But how? "No one knows for sure," says Dr. Resnick. "My theory is that supplemental calcium alters the hormones that help regulate blood pressure. But a lot more research needs to be done before we figure out exactly what's going on."

And more work *is* being done. In fact, Dr. Resnick's results have been corroborated by the investigators from Oregon Health Sciences University. They too found that oral calcium could lower blood pressure, but at a much lower dose.

For eight weeks they gave 1,000 milligrams of calcium or a placebo (inactive pill) to 70 patients, some with high blood pressure and some without. As expected, the nutrient pulled pressures down—in 42 percent of the hypertensives and 13 percent of those with normal pressures. And what's just as significant, none of the patients had to stop the calcium supplements because of side effects (*Clinical Research,* vol. 32, no. 1, 1984).

"These results," the researchers say, "suggest that long-term oral calcium may be effective nonpharmacologic [nondrug] therapy for reducing a subset of hypertensives' blood pressure and may also reduce blood pressure in selected normals [nonhypertensives]."

This may prove to be especially compelling news for pregnant women, and the reason is preeclampsia, a disorder arising in expectant mothers (6 to 7 percent of pregnant women in the United States) that causes 100 to 125 American fetal deaths a day. Its chief symptom: high blood pressure. Thus, researchers have asked the inevitable question of whether calcium—the antihypertensive—can counterpunch preeclampsia.

For answers, researchers have studied large populations and come up with some thought-provoking facts.

Jose Villar, M.D., of Johns Hopkins University in Baltimore, and his colleagues examined the incidence of eclampsia (preeclampsia's more serious form) and nutrient intake in Guatemala, Colombia and the United States. They discovered that low calcium intake consistently accompanied eclampsia, and vice versa. Guatemala had low eclampsia incidence and high calcium intake. Cali, Colombia, showed high incidence and low intake. The United States had low incidence and high intake. And the differences in incidence, say the researchers, had little to do with the age of the pregnant women or the prenatal care they got (*International Journal of Gynecology and Obstetrics,* vol. 21, 1983).

Perhaps more to the point, Dr. Villar and his colleagues have actually tested calcium's effect on blood pressure in pregnant women. They selected 36 healthy expectant mothers and during the second and third trimesters gave them daily doses of 1,000 milligrams of calcium, 2,000 milligrams of calcium, or a placebo. They monitored the women's blood pressure every step of the way.

When the data were compiled, it was clear that the supplemented women fared far better than the placebo group. Compared to the unsupplemented women, those taking 1,000 milligrams of calcium had reduced systolic pressure in the second trimester, and those on 2,000 milligrams had lower pressure throughout most of the study (*American Journal of Obstetrics and Gynecology,* May 15, 1983).

"Based on what we now know about eclampsia and hypertension in pregnancy," says Dr. Villar, "we recommend that all pregnant women at least meet their calcium RDA of 1,200 milligrams a day."

And judging from the current boom in calcium research, the calcium lessons in high school health class may never be the same.

Protecting and Restoring Your Good Health

Ease Your Blood Pressure Down Naturally

You begin your day with a juicy half-moon of cantaloupe, a glass of freshly squeezed orange juice and a bowl of bran cereal with a half cup of skim milk.

Lunch is broiled mackerel, parsley potatoes and a side salad of watercress, carrot medallions and almonds, tossed with your own dressing made of fresh garlic in corn oil and apple-cider vinegar.

Midafternoon, you calm your rumbling stomach with a cup of low-fat yogurt into which you've sliced half a banana.

For dinner, you whip up a luscious casserole of brown rice, onions, broccoli, cashews and melted part-skim mozzarella, lightly spiced with garlic.

If you have high blood pressure, theoretically you've just done everything right. Your one day's menu contains every nutrient known to *lower* blood pressure. Today, medical research has uncovered a way to fight hypertension that's more positive than just avoiding salt and saturated fat. There are actually foods you can eat more of that help you win this often-deadly numbers game.

And if you didn't know already, high blood pressure can be deadly. According to Michael Rees, M.D., author of *The Complete Family Guide to Living with High Blood Pressure* (Prentice-Hall, 1980), hypertension is the single most important cause of strokes, a major cause of diseases of the brain, kidneys and eyes and is the cause of an estimated one-third of all heart disease. Some 60 million Americans have blood pressures that are too high, blood pressures that might just respond to some dietary fine-tuning. They might want to start with the foods discussed here.

Cantaloupe, winter squash, potatoes, broccoli, orange juice, some fresh fruits, and milk.

These are foods containing hefty amounts of potassium. The fact is, how much potassium you have in your diet may be just as important as how little sodium you eat. Studies of vegetarians, who tend to have lower blood pressures than meat eaters, found that their sodium intake was no different from that of hypertensives but their potassium intake was significantly higher.

A group of scientists in Israel looked at the eating habits of 98 vegetarians whose average age was 60 and compared them to a similar group of meat eaters. What they found was a very low prevalence of hypertension—only 2 percent—among the vegetarians, although they lived in an adult population where the expected prevalence was 20 to 25 percent. The vegetarians ate as much salt as their neighbors and had the same genetic predisposition to developing hypertension. But they didn't. The researchers concluded that it was their potassium-rich diets of vegetables, fruits and nuts that kept them from developing hypertension (*American Journal of Clinical Nutrition,* May, 1983).

Just how does potassium protect the body from hypertension, even when sodium intake isn't restricted? No one really knows, although there are a number of theories. For one, potassium is an effective diuretic—and has been used as one for nearly four centuries. But in addition to helping the body rid itself of water, potassium also helps slough off sodium, an effect called natriuresis. Potassium also appears to act on several important physiological systems that regulate blood pressure and control the workings of the vascular system.

In both animal and human studies, potassium seems to have little effect on people whose blood pressures are normal. But it can produce a significant drop in both systolic and diastolic pressures of hypertensives.

And there may be one group of people for whom potassium is literally a shield against the ravages of excess sodium. According to George R. Meneely, M.D., professor emeritus of medicine at Louisiana State University School of Medicine, there may be "a substantial fraction of the population worldwide, including primitive societies, who develop elevation of the blood pressure if they eat more than four grams of sodium as sodium chloride [normal table salt] a day.

"There is extensive animal evidence," says Dr. Meneely, "that the hypertensogenic [hypertension-causing] effect of excess sodium is counteracted by extra dietary potassium. There is pretty good literature on its effect in humans too."

For anyone who wants to increase his or her dietary potassium, here's a cooking tip from a group of Swedish scientists: To avoid potassium loss in cooking, steam rather than boil vegetables. When doctors at a Swedish hospital tested the two cooking methods with potatoes, a rich source of potassium, they discovered that boiled potatoes lost 10 to 50 percent of their potassium while steamed potatoes lost only 3 to 6 percent. They had similar results with carrots, beans and peas (*Lancet,* January 15, 1983).

Dairy products, leafy green vegetables like kale and watercress, and nuts. If you've been scrupulous about cutting sodium out of your diet, you may be cutting out calcium, too. There's a convincing amount of evidence from all corners of the world indicating calcium can lower your blood pressure. Unfortunately, the best sources of calcium—dairy products—also have a fair amount of sodium. A two-ounce serving of Swiss cheese contains 544 milligrams of calcium (the Recommended Dietary Allowance, or RDA, is 800 milligrams), but there's a hefty 148 milligrams of sodium in there, too. But the evidence is too overwhelming in favor of calcium as an antidote to hypertension for anyone to give up milk and cheese entirely.

Consider, for example, a study of 82 percent of the adult residents of Rancho Bernardo, an upper-middle-class community in Southern California. What separated the male hypertensives from the normotensives, according to researchers at the University of California in San Diego, was milk. Milk consumption was lower in borderline, untreated and treated hypertensives (*American Journal of Clinical Nutrition,* September, 1983).

In an even larger study involving 20,749 people across the country, calcium was the only one of 17 nutrients evaluated that differed in the hypertensives. Those people with high blood pressure consumed 18 percent less calcium (*Annals of Internal Medicine,* May, 1983).

That figure alarms researcher David McCarron, M.D., of the division of nephrology and hypertension at the Oregon Health Sciences University in Portland. He conducted that particular study—and several others linking calcium and blood pressure—and he's convinced that a good hypertensive diet has to contain dairy products, sodium and cholesterol notwithstanding.

"If you have to, switch to low-sodium or low-cholesterol cheeses, which are an excellent source of calcium and low in saturated fatty acids," he says. "If you don't have a cholesterol problem and you're near your ideal body weight, you don't necessarily have to worry about the cholesterol."

As for sodium, Dr. McCarron's work indicates that calcium may actually negate the harmful effects of salt on the system. An increased calcium load tends to facilitate the body's excretion of sodium, he notes.

Nuts, brown rice, molasses, milk, wheat germ, bananas, potatoes and soy products. Inadequate dietary magnesium has been shown to increase blood pressure in both animals and humans. Though the exact mechanism isn't known, there is some indication that magnesium exerts its pressure-lowering effect by regulating the entry and exit of calcium in the smooth muscle cells of the vascular system. Together, the two minerals produce the regular contraction and relaxation of blood vessels.

In a test involving untreated, newly diagnosed hypertensives, Dr. McCarron found that they consumed less calcium and magnesium than a similar group whose blood pressures were normal. Sodium intake didn't seem to matter (*Annals of Internal Medicine,* May, 1983).

"The interaction of magnesium and calcium gives the calcium the ability to get where it has to in a cell," says Dr. McCarron. "Magnesium facilitates calcium getting to the right place where it can have this relaxing effect."

Polyunsaturated fats.
In a pilot study of healthy people in Italy, Finland and the United States, researchers discovered that the level of dietary linoleic acid—polyunsaturated fats—was associated with incidence of high blood pressure. There were more hypertensives among the Finnish population than among the Italians and Americans. The Finns consumed more saturated and less polyunsaturated fats than the others.

When a group of Finns aged 40 to 50 were placed on a low-fat diet high in polyunsaturated fats and low in saturated fats, even when salt consumption wasn't reduced, blood pressures dropped significantly. When they turned to their old eating habits, their old blood pressures returned, too (*American Journal of Clinical Nutrition,* December, 1983).

What's the magic? James M. Iacono, Ph.D., and other researchers at the U.S. Department of Agriculture Western

Human Nutrition Research Center in San Francisco, have one theory. They believe polyunsaturated fats lower blood pressure because, when they're metabolized by the body, they yield a substance that is essential for making prostaglandins. These are fatty acids that seem to control pressure by aiding in the sloughing off of water and salt from the kidneys (*Hypertension,* September/October, 1982).

Mackerel and other marine fish high in eicosapentanoic acid, one of the omega-3 fatty acids.

Tests in Germany involving 15 volunteers on a mackerel diet provided some heartening results. After only two weeks, serum triglycerides and total cholesterol dropped significantly, mirrored by "markedly lower" systolic and diastolic blood pressures.

The Germans didn't simply pull mackerel out of their hats. They were attempting to approximate the diet of Greenland Eskimos and Japanese fishermen, who enjoy a very low incidence of cardiovascular disease. The key appears to be the omega-3 fatty acids found in many fish (*Atherosclerosis,* volume 49, 1983).

Another study tested the effects of cod-liver oil on the Western diet. Cod-liver oil also contains omega-3 fatty acids. A group of volunteers added three tablespoons of cod-liver oil a day to their normal diets and wound up with lower blood pressures (*Circulation,* March, 1983).

Bran, fresh fruit and vegetables, beans and whole grain breads.

The factor here is fiber. There are some early indications from recent tests that plant fiber can significantly lower blood pressure, though precisely why is still a mystery.

Researcher James W. Anderson, M.D., of the Veterans Administration Medical Center in Lexington, Kentucky, placed 12 diabetic men on a 14-day diet containing more than three times the dietary fiber (and fat) of a control diet. Average blood pressures dropped 10 percent. In patients whose blood pressures had been normal, systolic pressures were 8 percent lower and diastolic figures dropped 10 percent.

The news was even better for the men who had high blood pressures to begin with. Their systolic pressures dropped by 11 percent and diastolic pressures by 10 percent (*Annals of Internal Medicine,* May, 1983).

Dr. Anderson was pleased with his results, but he's not sure why he got them. "My strongest hunch is that it's related to certain changes in insulin. The patients' insulin needs were low on the high-fiber diet. There's a lot of evidence that insulin contributes to high blood pressure. It's basically a salt-retentive hormone. We also reported in a small increase in sodium loss in feces. I didn't think at the time it was meaningful but thinking about it later, having two different mechanisms working together like that—the insulin and the sodium excretion—you can get a synergistic effect."

What makes the results even more significant is that salt use was not restricted during the diet. "In fact," says Dr. Anderson, "there was a 50 percent increase in sodium intake. But potassium also went up, so the sodium:potassium ratio stayed the same."

High Blood Pressure? Take a Second Look!

8:30 A.M. Tea and toast with the missus. Blood pressure 118/77.

11:10 A.M. Son calls to say he has joined obscure religious sect. B.P. 130/85.

2:30 P.M. Called into boss's office to discuss new computer system and possibility of early retirement. B.P. 145/90.

6 P.M. Lite beer in La-Z-Boy. Dog brings slippers. B.P. 125/83.

10 P.M. Reading *War and Peace* before bed. B.P. 120/79.

Most of us speak of our blood pressure the same way we do our shoe size, as a fixed figure—120/80 if we're "normal," higher or lower if we're not. The figure we cite is usually a single reading taken in a doctor's office. We are sitting, possibly chatting with the doctor or nurse, and are probably nervous. But recently developed lightweight automatic blood-pressure cuffs have made it possible to monitor your blood pressure 24 hours a day, even while you sleep. And these readings have confirmed something we suspected all along. Blood pressure varies tremendously, not just with our body's natural cycles of temperature, hormone secretion, waking and sleeping, but particularly in response to our feelings, actions and environment.

A newborn baby's pressure may double when it begins to cry. And when adults cry, or laugh, their blood pressure first peaks, then begins a sustained and soothing decline. Our pressure drops when we pat a dog or gaze at an aquarium full of fish. It is lower when it is taken by a nurse than by a doctor, and it tends to drop slightly in each of a series of readings. It rises when we talk, shovel snow, defecate or make love. Weight lifters experience the ultimate in high blood pressure, up to 450/300, apparently with no ill effects.

"What *doesn't* our blood pressure respond to?" asks Franz Halberg, M.D., a professor at the University of Minnesota and coiner of the term "circadian rhythm."

In studies involving repeated, long-term monitoring of a number of women, Dr. Halberg found that both systolic and diastolic blood pressure varied by an average of 40 millimeters of mercury daily—much more than what most people think of as an average range. And occasionally he found as much as a 100-point spread between a woman's sleeping blood pressure and her pressure under stress.

Yearly changes in blood pressure also occurred, in relationship to the blood level of a hormone called aldosterone, which is secreted by the adrenal gland and affects blood volume through our body's retention of sodium and excretion of potassium. Aldosterone was slightly higher in winter and lower in summer, and women who had other indications of being at high risk for cardiovascular disease had less yearly change in aldosterone level, Dr. Halberg says.

Another ongoing study involving 17,000 people in England found blood pressure slightly higher in winter than in summer, and the effects of seasonal change greater in older than in younger subjects. These researchers attribute the increase to vascular constriction during cold weather. They note an almost 50 percent increase in sudden heart attacks and strokes during the winter, and up to a 70 percent increase during extremely cold weather (*British Medical Journal,* October 2, 1982).

But by far the biggest changes in blood pressure come in response to our interaction with our environment. This response is complex. Certainly it involves both automatic and learned behavior. It probably includes adrenaline production, in response to sudden noises or crazed taxi drivers, for instance, as part of our body's primitive "fight or flight" response. But it also includes all of modern man's worries, expectations and lifestyle— even our self-image and ability to express our emotions.

These changes are particularly fascinating to researchers because they seem to be something people can learn to control if they are taught healthy new ways to respond to stress.

Talking, for instance, even about such impersonal topics as the weather, can be such a blood pressure elevator that researchers at the University of Maryland say hypertension can be influenced as much by problems surrounding communication as it can by being overweight.

"Communication is very important to our bodies," says James Lynch, Ph.D., of the university's Psychophysiological Clinic. "One of the leading causes of premature death in this country is loneliness, and that is why communication is so vital. But it can be a major source of stress."

Dr. Lynch has found that when a normal person speaks, his blood pressure rises 10 to 20 percent above its usual baseline pressure. And in a hypertensive person, pressure can rise as much as 50 percent. People with high blood pressure often unconsciously hold their breath when they speak, and speak rapidly when they are excited, he adds.

His colleague, clinic director Sue Ann Thomas, R.N., Ph.D., noticed that many hypertensives seem to be out of touch with their bodies and their feelings—not recognizing such physical signs of stress as muscle tension, increased respiration and pulse rate. They seem oblivious to the things in their life producing the stress.

"The things people react to most physiologically are things

they are cognitively unaware of," Dr. Thomas says. "One man might come in and say his mother-in-law raises his blood pressure, and when he talks about her, his blood pressure might go up somewhat. But the changes are not as significant as when he talks about his son being in jail for the third time. Yet that might be something he says he is *not* concerned about, because there is nothing he can do about it."

Their program for hypertensives is designed to make a graphic, undeniable connection between a person's skyrocketing blood pressure and a specific stressor, and to teach people to break that connection.

A patient is hooked up to an automatic monitor that flashes his blood pressure on a screen every minute. Then, he and a therapist began to probe for issues and areas in his life that are raising his blood pressure. The patient can see the physiological response and slowly begins to recognize the physical symptoms of stress. At the same time, he also learns how to react less to a stressful subject. He is taught to talk more slowly and to take deep breaths while talking, and to stop to listen.

As patients gain control over this technique, Dr. Thomas says, "We point out to them, 'Look, you really *do* have a choice. You *can* choose not to have your blood pressure go up so much.'" Part of the therapy also involves making people more flexible in their standards and getting them to see the humor in life. "These people really want things to go well, and they are furious when they don't. They also tend to get serious very quickly. We show them how much a laugh can lower their blood pressure," Dr. Thomas says.

Milt Soskin, a Philadelphia businessman, found his blood pressure dropped from about 165/95 to 128/76 on the program. Always a loud and fast talker, Soskin says his only real therapy was to learn to speak calmly. A happy fringe benefit has been a better relationship with his family and friends. "I could never listen. Now I do." Even his employees have benefited. "I had a meeting this morning with some of my key executives, and with me as leader speaking slowly and quietly, everyone else speaks more slowly and quietly. It is a calmer atmosphere and we get more work done."

Soskin admits he was prone to a lot of self-induced anxiety, much of it about his business. But you don't have to be president of your own company to react to work.

Indeed—and just what we all wanted to hear—working may be hazardous to our health, according to the findings of Thomas Pickering, M.D., associate professor of medicine at Cornell University Medical Center.

Dr. Pickering's around-the-clock monitoring of several hundred people has shown their pressures to be highest at work—up to 10 points more than their 24-hour baseline reading, even though they had sedentary jobs. On days off, their blood pressure did not show this elevation. And people who tended to have higher baseline blood pressure had a greater increase in pressure at work than people with normal blood pressure.

"Our present feeling is that blood pressure at work may be the most important pressure to monitor," Dr. Pickering says. "It is the people who have high blood pressure at work who tend to have cardiovascular disease. Work is the form of stress people are most regularly exposed to."

Dr. Pickering also found the doctor's office a disturbing place.

While people with normal blood pressure had slightly lower readings in the doctor's office than at home, people diagnosed as true hypertensives or as borderline had their highest readings of the day in the doctor's office, about 10 points over their 24-hour average. The jump was apparently the result of the anxiety they were feeling over having their blood pressure taken and the fear that it would be high.

Unfortunately, this "defense reaction," as Dr. Pickering calls it, could become a vicious cycle that leads to a misdiagnosis and possible unnecessary treatment for high blood pressure. "People who have been found to have high blood pressure once are usually told to have it checked again. They become even more anxious the second time the reading is taken, their blood pressure goes up and the diagnosis is 'confirmed,' and it just goes on from there," Dr. Pickering says.

In fact, he says the main practical implication of his study is that in patients with mild hypertension (a diastolic reading between 90 and 104), clinic readings may give a misleading impression of overall blood pressure. In these patients, Dr. Pickering says, a 24-hour reading may be particularly helpful.

New Natural Approaches to Sciatica

When the pain struck, hairdresser Sharon Brown exhausted every medical option she could think of, from aspirin to orthopedic surgeons to chiropractors. But the pain didn't go away. She did find out it had a name. The doctors called it sciatica, and told her she was in its "later stages."

"One doctor told me I'd probably have to have surgery and that it still might not go away. Then he told me to stay off my feet. In my business? Then, do you know what he said? He said, 'I hope I'm not scaring you.' Scaring me? I was in the later stages of berserk!"

But Sharon Brown didn't take surgery for an answer. She shopped around until she found a chiropractor who took her pain away through intermittent traction. "He said I didn't need to come back unless it started hurting again," she says. "I've felt fine ever since."

Sciatica. It's a symptom its sufferers elevate to a disease, a laming pain that starts in the lower back and radiates down the leg, sometimes bringing with it a cold numbness. Specifically, it's an irritation of the sciatic nerve, the largest nerve in the body. And once you track its pathway, you begin to understand the vast geography of sciatica's pain.

The roots of the sciatic nerve are in the pelvis. From there it runs through the buttocks and the back of the thigh, splitting into two nerves just above the back of the knee and skimming in tandem down the leg to the foot. An injury, even the slightest pressure anywhere along the lengthy nerve line, can trigger a debilitating sciatica attack.

Sometimes it takes sophisticated equipment to track down the cause, which can be as simple as a muscle spasm or as serious as a tumor. On rare occasions, it's less baffling. In one case reported several years ago in the *Journal of the American Medical Association*, the patient's sciatica was traced to an overly flat wallet he carried in his rear pocket. The "ailment" was relieved immediately when he switched to a coat pocket, a procedure his physician called a "wallectomy."

It is not rare for sciatica to heal spontaneously. It is also common for a cure to be difficult to conjure up. Like Sharon Brown, most victims have to comparison shop for the treatment that works for them. They may have to experiment with techniques as varied as acupressure and hot baths—and combinations thereof—before they come up with the right prescription for their pain.

It may take time, and the cure may not be permanent, but the search is not going to be fruitless, says Lawrence Friedmann, M.D., coauthor of *Freedom from Backaches* (Simon & Schuster). "Not all headaches are relieved by aspirin, nor all disease germs overcome by penicillin," he says. "No treatment is effective for all. Certainly there is no single treatment effective for all cases of backache—yet, almost invariably, some way can be found to relieve backache."

With that optimistic prognosis, where do you start? With a good diagnosis, the doctors say.

"The first thing you need is an adequate medical and neurological examination," says Howard D. Kurland, M.D., a psychiatrist and neurologist, and the author of *Back Pains— Quick Relief without Drugs* (Simon & Schuster, 1981). "You have to make sure it's not some disease or disorder that needs something other than symptomatic treatment."

The most common cause of sciatica is the proverbial bad back. It could be a herniated disk, injury to the cushionlike ring of cartilage and connective tissue that sits between the vertebrae of the spine. These disks are what give our spines mobility, allowing us to twist and turn and bend. Years of wear and tear or a sudden injury can damage a disk, causing the soft, gelatinous core to ooze out and press against the nerve roots that thread through the spinal column, telegraphing pain along the lengthy course of the nerve.

Sometimes the only cure for this painful condition is surgery. But sometimes it needs no treatment at all because the protruding disk nucleus is severed and drops off harmlessly or slides back into the disk if the pressure that caused it to pop out is relieved by bed rest.

"Nobody ever died from not having surgery on their back," says Milton Fried, M.D., an Atlanta physician with a rare pedigree—he is also a chiropractor. "I'd say I send 1 of 5,000 patients for surgery. Except for rare conditions where the spinal cord could be involved, surgery should absolutely not be considered as an early treatment."

One reason is the high rate of spontaneous recovery. The other is that a herniated disk is only one of "50 or more possible causes of sciatica," according to Dr. Friedmann.

"You could have what we call a pseudodisk problem," he says. "The sciatic nerve can be irritated by a muscle spasm that puts pressure on the nerve. You can hit the sciatic nerve somewhere in the back of the leg and produce the same type of pain."

If you've had the more serious possibilities ruled out, you can test yourself for muscle spasm (with the help of a friend), says Dr. Friedmann. Muscle spasms tend to leave muscles tender to the touch. Your examiner should use the heel of his hands or his fingertips and gently knead the muscles of your back like pastry dough until he discovers the tender center of pain.

What caused the muscle spasm in the first place could be a thornier mystery to untangle. It could be anything from an injury to tension, says Dr. Friedmann. But in all likelihood, he says, the bottom line is a loss of elasticity and strength of the muscles that support the back, including the abdominals. "In 81 percent of the patients I see with back problems, it's due to this loss of elasticity and strength," the physician says. "You get muscle pain and spasm, which itself gives you back pain and radiating pain, because you've asked your muscles to exceed their ability."

Weak stomach muscles, in fact, may trigger the chain of events that leads to this overtaxing of the back muscles, injury and sciatica. Dr. Friedmann notes that researchers at the State University of Iowa College of Medicine discovered that the abdominal muscles of chronic backache patients were less than a third as strong as their back muscles. In that study and others, "very often strengthening of abdominal muscles proved to be all that was necessary to eliminate backaches," says Dr. Friedmann.

Regular exercise is not only a therapy but a preventive, he

says. But it's a long-term solution, not meant to bring on fast relief. Is there anything short of surgery and drugs that will bring calm and peace to your sciatic nerve? Dr. Kurland thinks so. So does Michael Reed Gach, author of *The Bum Back Book* (Acu Press, 1983). Both advocate the use of acupressure, a needleless form of acupuncture that relieves pain with the firm touch of a finger.

No one is really sure why acupuncture works, but it does, says Dr. Kurland. "I know it does because I have seen it work on hundreds of patients and felt it work on myself," says the physician, himself a backache sufferer. What science does know is that many of the 500 or more acupuncture points lie along nerve pathways. There is a theory that the nervous system has "gates" that control the transmission of pain impulses to the brain and that acupuncture works by closing these gates, says Dr. Kurland.

Whatever the actual mechanism, for some people acupuncture is the answer to their pained prayers.

Acupressure works in much the same way as acupuncture, relieving pain by putting pressure on a point that may be far removed from its origin.

Dr. Kurland used the acupuncture points when developing his own auto-acupressure system, locating the nerve branches close enough to the skin to respond to the pressure of a thumbnail.

Accuracy is important in auto-acupressure, says Dr. Kurland. You have to score a direct hit for it to be effective. In general, you'll know because an acupressure point is more sensitive to the pressure than the areas surrounding it. When you locate it, you should feel a tingling sensation, as if you had just hit your funny bone, says the physician.

There are two points that may help relieve sciatica. The first is found at the top of the buttocks, between the bone that anchors the spine to the pelvic girdle and the large knob near the end of the thighbone. To find it, stand up and put the heel of your hand on your hipbone with the fingers extending down the side of your leg. When you move your leg back and forth, you feel the large bony knob moving.

Now, lie down on your left side with your knees drawn up

comfortably. Find the bony knob again, then slide your thumb around until you find a large, flat prominence between the base of the spine and the tailbone. Estimate the distance between the two points. The point you want to stimulate is close to the knob, about a third of the distance between the knob and the flat area. Wrap the fingers around the thigh bone, using the thumb to apply enough pressure on the point to cause it to hurt. Hold for 30 seconds.

The second point is easier to find. The calf of the leg is shaped by a long muscle, anchored at the lower end by the Achilles tendon. Above that, it divides into two bands of "heads." You can feel a groove between the two heads, exactly in the middle of the calf at its widest point. This second point is at the lower end of the muscle groove. To stimulate it, put the nail of your bent thumb in the point and apply opposing pressure with your fingers on your shinbone. Hold for 30 seconds.

Other Home Remedies

There are other nonmedicinal, noninvasive relief methods, many of which you can do at home with a good measure of safety. "There should be no hesitation in using home remedies," says Dr. Friedmann. "The only danger is to rely on them entirely for relief of pain without getting to the cause of the pain."

Heat ● This will be especially helpful if the sciatica is caused by muscle spasm, says Dr. Friedmann. Wet or dry heat should be applied for 20 to 30 minutes at least twice a day, he says. A hot tub bath that lasts half an hour can be very soothing.

Massage ● Believe it or not, this is a form of exercise, albeit passive, says Dr. Friedmann. Although its great value may be in its calming effect on the psyche, there is evidence that a gentle massage can stimulate the nervous system, which in turn sparks the respiratory and circulatory systems to pump more healing blood and oxygen to the muscles. A massage actually can help relieve a tight muscle spasm. For a good home massage, Dr. Friedmann suggests an unscented talc or mineral oil as a lubricant. The person giving the massage should begin by lightly massaging the buttocks with the heel of the hand and work up each side of the spinal column without pressing on any bones.

Traction • The theory behind traction is simple. The gentle, constant pull allows the muscles to relax and joint structure to stretch. Often, joints are more properly aligned and pop back into the right place when the traction is stopped. Dr. Friedmann uses as much as 200 pounds of weight in intermittent traction on his patients. But home traction should be used only on the advice of a doctor, he cautions. Pelvic and cervical traction equipment is available at most surgical supply stores and pharmacies.

Lifestyle Change • How you stand, sit, sleep and bend and how much you weigh play a large role in the health of your back. Dr. Kurland has several tips for changing your lifestyle to spare yourself the pain of sciatica.

Weight—If you're overweight, you're putting abnormal stress on your spine. If you are prone to back problems, stick as close as possible to your ideal weight.

Sitting—Pick a straight-backed chair and sit with your knees higher than your hips because it puts less strain on your spine. When driving, sit close enough to the steering wheel so that you can keep your knees as high as possible.

Standing—To put the least strain on your back, try to rest one foot higher than the other. If you're in a situation where you can't, keep your back straight by tilting your pelvis or bend one knee, keeping the other knee straight.

Bending and Lifting—Most people know that the proper way to bend to pick something up is with the knees as well as the back, letting the legs do most of the work. If you are carrying something heavy, clutch it close to the body with the elbows bent. Try not to lift heavy objects in a tight, awkward place without help.

Sleeping—Any backache sufferer knows it's painful to lie on the stomach. The semifetal position—on the side with the knees and hips bent—is easiest on the back. Firm, flat mattresses are best. A California study found that waterbeds also are helpful to some chronic backache sufferers.

Manipulation ● Another alternative, although a controversial one, is spinal manipulation. Manipulation involves the actual moving of the bones of the spine to adjust them in their relationship to one another. It can be particularly helpful to sciatica sufferers if their pain is caused by a dislocated joint, says Dr. Friedmann. Manipulation can stretch the tissue that supports the joint to unlock the joint and snap it back into place. It can also help if the cause is a herniated disk, because it can break off the pulpy disk core that's pressing on the nerve. But, warns Dr. Friedmann, manipulation can also exacerbate that particular problem.

Dr. Fried, who uses manipulation, cautions against regarding it as a panacea, as many sufferers do. "It is not a cure-all," he says. "But it does have a definite place in the treatment of low back pain. It definitely helps some people, who walk into the chiropractor's office all doubled over and leave it walking straight. And it's a safe treatment, despite claims to the contrary. And it's a lot safer than surgery."

But, cautions Dr. Fried, make sure the practitioner you choose does a set of diagnostic x-rays before starting manipulative therapy to rule out more serious conditions, such as cancer, which can manifest themselves as low back pain.

How to Kill a Cold

Dr. M., a microbiologist and science fiction buff, recently treated his wife and kids to the latest special-effects fantasy film. Huddled together in the dark, sharing boxes of popcorn, they watched three zany young men chase green balls of protoplasm all over New York City, zapping them with a weapon no one had ever seen before: a ghostbuster.

After the movie, the family (unwisely) stopped off for deep-pan pizza (with anchovies) and later that night Dr. M. slept fitfully. Tossing and turning he imagined himself chasing little green micro-organisms all over town, zapping them with a weapon that to him was even more exciting than a ghostbuster: It was a *virus buster.*

Such is the stuff that dreams are made of. But in the real world of hospitals and laboratories, it would be a rare microbiologist who has never yearned for a virus buster of his own. Indeed, medical researchers and clinicians of all kinds have spent entire careers looking for weapons to use against these tiny, elusive goblins that persistently haunt us with colds, flu, herpes, shingles, hepatitis and more. The average American, says the U.S. Public Health Service, experiences more than 200 viral infections during his or her lifetime.

There are vaccines against a few of the scarier viruses—polio, for example, and measles—but there has never been a universal vaccine against colds and flu. Which means that it's time to take stock of the natural virus busters that we have at our disposal.

One of them is zinc. It's long been recognized that zinc in the diet is necessary for a strong immune response. Without zinc, the body's germ-fighting white blood cells would malfunction and wounds wouldn't heal. But a group of researchers in Austin, Texas, recently reported that zinc lozenges, dissolved in the mouth, can have a remarkably direct effect on the duration of colds.

This story actually begins three years ago, when an Austin urban planner, George A. Eby, gave zinc tablets to his then three-year-old daughter, who was fighting leukemia. He felt it would help boost her immunity. The little girl also suffered from severe colds which were coming at her one right after the other. Nothing dramatic happened until, on one occasion, the child decided to dissolve a 50-milligram zinc gluconate tablet in her mouth instead of swallowing it. Within hours, her cold symptoms vanished.

At Eby's request, his family physician and medical researchers at the Clayton Foundation Biochemical Institute in Austin set up an experiment to see whether zinc lozenges could cure other people's colds. Sixty-five people with colds took part in the experiment. Thirty-seven were given zinc gluconate tablets every other waking hour, and the rest received a harmless placebo. Each subject carefully recorded his or her headaches, sneezes and coughs for a week.

The results were almost too good to be true. "In the

zinc-treated group, sizable numbers of subjects became asymptomatic within hours," the researchers report. Within a day, one-fifth of the zinc group was fully recuperated. None of the placebo group recovered that fast. The average length of a cold was 3.9 days in the zinc group, compared to 10.8 days in the placebo group (*Antimicrobial Agents and Chemotherapy,* January, 1984).

But the zinc worked only when it was dissolved like a hard candy instead of being swallowed like a pill. That's because the zinc ions possibly came into direct contact with the viruses in the respiratory tract.

"We think that zinc inhibits the cleavage of viral polypeptides," says Donald R. Davis, Ph.D., of the Clayton Foundation, who analyzed the experiment. This polypeptide cleavage takes place inside a healthy cell which the virus has "hijacked," and cleavage must occur before a virus can clone itself. Zinc ions, however, may disrupt this process.

"We hope this will be a big step toward controlling the common cold," Dr. Davis says. "The next step is to find out exactly how much zinc should be used and how often it needs to be applied.

"You have to remember that we're talking about treating an existing cold, not preventing one," he adds. "Although it's possible that if your diet is rich in zinc, you would suffer fewer colds."

The zinc treatment comes with a few caveats, Dr. Davis admits. Several people dropped out of his experiment because they didn't like the taste of the lozenges. And not all zinc supplements are equally effective. In fact, Dr. Davis notes that the zinc treatment needs much further study before it can be recommended to the public.

Vitamin C and interferon are two more virus busters. There has been so much talk about synthesizing interferon and marketing it as a drug that we tend to forget that it is also a natural substance which protects us against invaders 24 hours a day without costing us a cent.

Whenever a healthy cell comes under attack by a virus, the cell manufacturers interferon and then sends it off in all directions like an army of Paul Reveres, warning neighboring cells to defend themselves.

Once a nearby cell is merely touched by interferon, it becomes incapable of doing what the virus most wants it to do—namely, to convert its nucleus into a virus factory. A cell that's immunized by interferon may still be invaded by a virus, but no new viruses will be born. To borrow computer terminology, the virus will be unable to replace the cell's genetic software with its own.

All cells have the ability to produce interferon, but we can give that ability a boost by increasing our intake of vitamin C. Benjamin Siegel, Ph.D., a professor of pathology at the Oregon Health Sciences University, has found that mice given vitamin C supplements have higher levels of interferon in their blood than mice who receive no extra vitamin C. "It's possible that vitamin C stimulates the increased production of interferon by the affected cell," he says. He takes 1,000 milligrams of vitamin C a day.

The body has another built-in virus buster: fever. Both flu viruses and cold viruses like it relatively cool. They flourish where the temperature is between 86° and 95° F. The body core is too hot for them, but the nasal passages, cooled by inhalation, are just right. Heat up the nostrils with fever, however, and the viruses shrivel up and die.

Here's how fever works. When viruses or bacteria invade the body, the germ-fighting white blood cells release a protein called pyrogen, a Greek word that means "heat-producing." Pyrogen tells the brain to raise the body's temperature from 98.6° to about 102° F. Experiments with animals have shown that when the temperature in the body goes up, the number of live viruses in the nasal passages goes down.

Fever is difficult to control, however, so other methods for heating up the nose and throat have been suggested. A steam bath followed by a hot toddy is one traditional cure. Inhaling warm water vapor is another. There is even a product on the market in Europe called a Rhinotherm, which shoots two jets of gentle steam into the nostrils.

Physical exercise is perhaps the most natural warm-up of all. One researcher has suggested that regular exercise promotes the release of pyrogen, which keeps the body temperature high for several hours after the workout is over (*Physician and Sportsmedicine,* March, 1983).

Not all virus busters, however, involve the help of nutrients or subcellular proteins. If we made a list of everything that fights viruses, that list would have to include companionship. People who have friends they can turn to in times of stress have more resistance to viral infections than people who are lonely.

In England a few years ago, a group of psychologists wanted to find what effect, if any, the emotional events in a person's life might have on the severity of their colds. Would a man's head cold, for instance, be worse if his love affair had just ended? Would a woman's cold be milder if she'd just gotten a new job? The psychologists had a hunch that emotional lows go hand-in-hand with bad colds. But they weren't sure.

To find out, they recruited 52 men and women between the ages of 18 and 49. They were housewives, students, working people and professionals. Each one went through a battery of psychological tests and personality inventories. How introverted or extroverted were they? Had they been seeing a lot of people lately or had they gone off by themselves? How were they spending their leisure time?

Then came the ultimate sacrifice. Each volunteer agreed to "catch a cold." They were all inoculated with common cold viruses and then confined to a hospital ward for 10 days of close observation. The amount of virus present in their mucus was precisely noted, as were their sneezes, coughs and even the number of tissues they used to blow their noses.

At its conclusion, the experiment yielded "clear evidence of a psychosomatic component in colds." People who were outgoing and extroverted had milder colds than people who were introverted. And it appeared that people who had recently withdrawn from their friends and hobbies had the worst cold symptoms of all.

But the clearest finding was that people who had gone through the most drastic life changes—either for the better or worse, it didn't seem to matter—had the highest virus levels in their respiratory tracts and therefore the worst infections (*Journal of Psychosomatic Research,* volume 24, 1980).

Loneliness and stress sometimes combine to put a double whammy on our resistance to viral infection. At Ohio State University, a group of researchers decided that they'd heard too many anecdotes about the way stress brings on herpes virus attacks, which produce cold sores and fever blisters. They wanted proof.

The researchers took three blood samples from a group of 49 medical students to determine the level of herpes virus antibodies in their blood. A high level of antibodies, in this case, would indicate a diminished resistance to the virus. Blood samples were taken a month before final exams, on the first day of final exams, and during the first week back from summer vacation. The students also took a psychological test to measure how lonely they were.

Resistance to the virus turned out to be highest after the vacation, when the students were relaxed. And the lonelier students had significantly less resistance to the virus than the more gregarious students had.

It's amazing how much confusion still exists about these minor viral infections that visit us year after year. John Mills, M.D., a professor of medicine and microbiology at the University of California School of Medicine in San Francisco, has taken the trouble to round up a few more tips on how to avoid cold and flu viruses.

• Colds are most often "caught" when someone rubs his or her nose or eye after having touched the hand of an infected person who has just touched his nose. Keeping hands away from noses is a good idea.

• Coughing and sneezing are definite signs of a cold, but they are much less likely to pass a cold from one person to another. Sneezes and coughs contain very little virus.

• Taking aspirin reduces the symptoms of a cold, but increases the amount of virus in the nose. If you take aspirin, be extra careful not to touch your nose.

• Merely rinsing your hands under water for 30 seconds effectively washes away any viruses that might be on them.

• Don't worry about venturing out into wintry weather. There's no evidence that cold weather alone will give you a virus infection or even worsen the one you may already have.

Help for Those
Aching Hip Joints

The hip is a fine example of form following function. It's a neatly designed ball-and-socket joint that can rotate millions of times without needing oiling or servicing, and can carry up to 15 times its normal load—more than a ton—before it collapses. It's the largest, most stable joint in the body. It's also one of the most stressed. What should surprise us is not that this masterpiece of evolutionary engineering doesn't always work perfectly, but that it works as well as it does.

In a healthy hip, the ball and socket are smoothly contoured and fit snugly together. Each is lined with a layer of rubbery cartilage that acts as an elastic cushion and, with proper lubrication, allows the ball to rotate smoothly in the socket.

The ball and socket are further joined together by sheets and strands of muscles and ligaments. The joint is also completely enclosed by a tough capsule of ligament tissue. This capsule is lined by a membrane that secretes a slippery liquid, called synovial fluid, into the space between the bones to lubricate the joint.

A hip that hurts isn't always easy to diagnose. The pain can come from injury to the joint itself, possibly caused by arthritis or a misaligned leg. It could be a lower back problem, with nerve pain radiating into the hip. It could be strained muscles or an inflamed bursa.

Many hip problems don't show up on x-rays, so it's up to doctors to use other methods, says Grant Lawton, M.D., a Salem, Oregon, orthopedic surgeon. To pinpoint a problem, doctors may check body alignment to see whether the back is curved or the pelvis tilted. They may test muscle strength and look for differences in leg length. They'll ask questions about exercise and work, and will check to see if more than one joint is affected.

Many people suffer from hip problems, but runners and dancers seem to get more than their share, mostly from strained muscles. So do parachutists, truck drivers and butchers. A parachutist who lands hard can ram his thighbone into the joint, causing serious damage. A truck driver can do the same thing braking his heavy rig, and the truck makes his leg vibrate, causing further damage. A butcher who walks and stands all day on cold concrete floors can have impact damage along with circulatory problems in his hip.

As one Florida doctor put it, "When you have hip pain, you have to look at everything."

Among older people, the most common cause of hip pain is simple wear and tear of the joint, called osteoarthritis or degenerative joint disease.

In this condition, the cartilage first softens and becomes pitted and frayed. It loses its elasticity and becomes more susceptible to further damage from stress. As the hip joint continues to degenerate, areas of cartilage may be worn away, allowing the bones to rub against each other.

"Most forms of arthritis cause an aching pain in the front of the hip, in the groin area," Dr. Lawton says. "At first the pain develops only after you've been on your leg for some time. As it progresses, people can bear their weight less time and walk shorter distances before the pain gets to the point where they have to stop and rest. At the end stage, people are in constant pain, even in bed at night. They will usually require hip replacement surgery."

Doctors distinguish between primary and secondary osteoarthritis. "In primary osteoarthritis, we really don't know what is causing the joint degeneration," Dr. Lawton says. "It could be a defect in the cartilage surface or, some researchers say, crystal deposits in the joint may lead to wear and tear."

In secondary osteoarthritis, on the other hand, doctors are able to identify a cause—an old injury, for instance, or a misalignment of the back or leg.

Although you might have recovered from a bad bump—maybe you were in a car accident and your knees slammed into the dashboard—these insults have left their mark on your hips. Such trauma can cause microfractures in the little calcium particles that make up the ball, or head, of the hip. When these fractures heal, extra calcium is laid down that stiffens and hardens the bone underneath the cartilage, making it less resilient, which means the cartilage must absorb more impact shock. Dislocations and other severe injuries can also damage cartilage, leaving it roughened and etched with tiny crevices. This irregular surface greatly accelerates wear-and-tear joint degeneration.

Body misalignments can cause hip pain in a number of ways. Sometimes a leg is out of line with the pelvis. "This may initially start out as a problem with flat feet, or with knock-knees, especially in overweight women," says Robert C. Bartlett, M.D., an Ocala, Florida, family practitioner and author of *Arthritis of the Hip: Yours and Mine* (Arcy Publishing Co.), which outlines his program for beating osteoarthritis. "The feet begin to bend in toward each other, then the knees do the same. The hips will then flay out. Any time the thighbone is out of alignment with the pelvis, more stress is put on the joint, which causes it to wear more quickly."

Runners whose feet tend to pronate (turn inward) may also have this problem.

Sometimes one leg is shorter than the other. "This is quite common, and I think it just reflects the fact that the right side of our body is not exactly like the left," Dr. Lawton says. It's the longer leg that gets the hip pain. When you walk, you push the ball of the thighbone up into the socket. With the longer leg, you do this harder, which makes it degenerate faster.

Often, a lift in the shoe of the shorter leg will alleviate this pain. "The general consensus among orthopedic surgeons is that any discrepancy of less than half an inch does not cause hip problems," Dr. Lawton says. "Over half an inch, though, and a lift is definitely indicated."

Often, what people call hip pain is not hip pain at all—it is back pain that is radiating into the pelvis or buttocks, Dr. Lawton says. The same pain pattern can stem from a variety of back problems—a ruptured disk, degenerate disk disease, muscle strains, twisting injuries. Stretched muscles and ligaments in the lower back can also cause pain around the hip.

"I have found that an exercise program to diminish the swayback that is so common with this sort of hip pain tends to resolve the majority of problems," Dr. Lawton says. In cases that don't respond well to exercise, he also suggests physical therapy or back manipulation by an osteopathic doctor.

Can running cause hip problems? "You bet," says William A. Grana, M.D., director of the Oklahoma Center for Athletes in Oklahoma City. "Running is a swift and sure way to aggravate a pre-existing hip condition you may not even know you have, such as an inherited instability of the joint or early cartilage damage."

Running is particularly unforgiving in beginning or weekend exercisers who may not have developed the strength in their pelvic muscles to protect their hips and lower back from constant pounding, Dr. Grana says. "Running will help to develop these muscles, but we recommend you get them in shape *before* you start."

Longtime runners have other relatively minor hip problems that can still cause quite a bit of pain, says John G. Paty Jr., M.D., an associate clinical professor at the University of Tennessee at Chattanooga. Dr. Paty is involved in a 20-year study of joint changes in long-distance runners.

Bursas, the lubrication fluid-filled sacs that help the muscles glide smoothly over bone surfaces, can become inflamed (a condition called bursitis) from abuse or overuse of muscles, Dr. Paty says. A large bursa just inches below the head of the thighbone, on the outside of the leg, covers a bony projection called the greater trochanter. This bursa can become irritated by overly tense muscles, running in a tight circle or on an uneven surface, and by repetitive leg lifts. This area will feel tender and sore, especially when you lie on that side. Rest, ice and ultrasound are prescribed, although sometimes the only long-term relief seems to be a corticosteroid injection into the bursa, Dr. Paty says. Stretching these outer leg muscles before you begin running can prevent problems.

An irritated sacroiliac, the joint that attaches the spine to the pelvis, can appear as hip pain. Repetitive pounding combined with the slight sway of the pelvis as you run, especially in women, seems to be enough to aggravate that joint in some people, Dr. Paty says.

Some doctors suspect long-term running can damage otherwise healthy joints. "There is some data in animals that shows it might, but it hasn't been proven yet in man," Dr. Paty says. Studies of people who have been running many years are flawed, he says, "because you are looking only at those who made it, not those who dropped out years ago because of pain. The question we want to answer is, 'Can you exceed the capacity of your joints by the kind of mileage we see people running week after week, year after year?' "

Both Dr. Paty and Dr. Grana suggest you run on a soft surface, wear good footgear, warm up first and pay heed to hip pain. "Running just isn't for everybody," Dr. Grana says. "We try to get people into swimming or biking. These activities are just as good for your heart and lungs without putting tremendous stress on your joints. And for older people, long, brisk walks can be a healthy substitute for running."

What else can you do for hip pain? Lose that excess weight, Dr. Bartlett says. "That's the first thing I tell people with bad hips. No matter what else they do they're not going to get anywhere until they get their weight down to a reasonable level."

Excess weight actually compresses the space between the bones in the hip joint, making friction between the ball and socket much more likely.

People with cartilage damage can benefit by keeping their weight off the hip joint, Dr. Bartlett says. "Forearm crutches can take off much of your body weight and extend the life of a hip seemingly destined for replacement surgery. They give the cartilage a chance to regenerate itself without being worn down. Of course, when you are 60 years old, that repairing power isn't as much as when you're younger, but there's still some there." He suggests the patient "swallow his pride" and use the crutches faithfully for a few months until the hip pain cools down, then switch to a cane part of the time. The cane, by the way, should always be used in the hand *opposite* the damaged joint.

Shock-absorbing shoes can also cushion the blow, Dr. Lawton says. "Soft, crepe-soled shoes or running shoes can make a big difference, especially when people are walking or standing on hard surfaces all day long.

"Posture certainly plays a major role in the hip pain caused by a back problem," Dr. Lawton says. Slouching and crossing your legs at the knee are both culprits. And standing with your weight on one leg can contribute to a bursitis problem by tightening the muscles on the outside of the leg.

Warm, moist heat—a hot, wet cloth or a soak in the tub—seems to work best to relieve hip pain, doctors agree. If heat doesn't work, try massaging the sore area with an ice cube.

Porous bones and weak connective tissues can aggravate a hip problem. In osteoporosis, bone growth around the hip socket actually increases, as the bone tries frantically to offset its losses elsewhere, Dr. Lawton says. This leads to a buildup of calcium around the edges of the joint—bone spurs that cause painful grating.

"Almost all my patients end up taking 1,000 milligrams of supplemental calcium and 400 milligrams of supplemental magnesium so that they're getting a total of 1,500 milligrams of calcium and 500 milligrams of magnesium a day," Dr. Lawton says.

"I think this is very important in any female over age 30 to help prevent osteoporosis."

For back-related hip pain, 1,000 to 2,000 milligrams of vitamin C seems to help some people get better faster and have less recurrent problems, Dr. Lawton says.

"Vitamin C is an important part of collagen formation and probably helps strengthen the covering around the disk. That's probably the primary reason for its benefit," he explains.

An Antistroke Program

Stroke is an exceedingly nasty word. So nasty, in fact, that for years American doctors avoided using it at all. It was good enough for the ancient Greeks, who coined the term *apoplexy*, or "to be struck down," and for the British, who translated apoplexy to *stroke*. But it wasn't until the 1950s that our doctors abandoned their long-standing euphemism for stroke—cerebrovascular accident—and started calling a spade a spade. Only salty old New Englanders seem to have ignored the change. They've always referred to strokes as "shocks."

By any name, though, it's impossible to paint a benign portrait of a disease that might best be described as a heart attack in the brain.

"Stroke is more a disabler than it is a killer," says Boston neurologist Philip A. Wolf, M.D. "It can take away everything from your command of language to your ability just to go to the bathroom alone. There are people who would rather die than have one."

To quickly define this illness: There are three basic kinds of stroke. The most common is the thrombotic stroke, in which arteries become so thickened with fatty deposits or plaque that blood can't reach the brain. Then there are embolic strokes, where bits of plaque break loose from diseased arterial walls, drift "upstream" and eventually block a blood vessel in the brain. Finally, there are hemorrhagic strokes, in which blood pressure rises to the point of bursting an artery like an old, rusty water main.

In each case, the brain cells that are deprived of blood either die or become inactive. When they do, the functions they control—speech, vision, movement—die with them.

What makes strokes so scary is that the neurological damage they cause cannot in most cases be repaired or reversed. On top of that, stroke isn't like an infectious disease that at least leaves it victims immune to reinfection. A stroke means that more strokes are likely in the future. Even ministrokes, or transient ischemic attacks (TIA), which cause temporary blindness or numbness, are predictors of more serious strokes to come.

This sense of finality has led most specialists to believe that prevention is the only practical treatment for stroke. If the "correctable" precursors of stroke—high blood pressure, heart disease, diabetes and high cholesterol level—can be prevented, then stroke can be prevented. The experts seem to concur on this.

"Stroke is eminently preventable," says Paul Whelton, M.D., of the Johns Hopkins School of Medicine in Baltimore. "It's not like other diseases that we *think* can be prevented. We're sure we know how to prevent strokes."

For one thing, it is clear that the stroke rate would decline sharply if everyone checked his own blood pressure regularly and took steps to reduce it if it was high. There are an estimated 37 million hypertensives (as those with the condition are called), and each one is a potential candidate for stroke. As many as 75 percent of all stroke victims are said to have high blood pressure, and controlling it has been called the "most important single measure in the prevention of stroke." Says Dr. Whelton, "We seldom see a stroke victim who hasn't had a history of high blood pressure. There's a very close relationship between the two."

How high is high? The now-famous Framingham study, in which the medical histories of the citizens of a small Massachusetts town have been monitored closely by neurologists, cardiologists and others for more than a generation, showed that blood pressure higher than 160/95 in men was often associated with the risk of stroke (*Stroke,* May/June, 1982).

Other studies have confirmed that blood pressure and stroke risk consistently rise together. In Finland, where high-fat dairy foods are dietary staples and cardiovascular disease is common, men with systolic blood pressure (the larger of the two numbers in a blood pressure reading) between 150 and 189 have twice the stroke risk of someone with less than 150, while men and women with systolic pressure above 190 carry four times and two times, respectively, the risk of the under-150 group (*Stroke,* May/June, 1982).

Changing to a healthier diet is one way to reduce both high blood pressure and the risk of stroke. Calcium, for instance, seems to help. Surveys have shown that the calcium intake of people with high blood pressure runs between 10 and 65 percent less than people with normal blood pressure. Eliminating salt and salty foods can decrease blood pressure, and giving up caffeine also helps, according to some studies.

Evidence that a high-fiber, low-sodium and low-fat diet can lower blood pressure was uncovered recently in England. In one particular study, 35 people with both high pressure and diabetes agreed to give up their customary high-fat, high-calorie "Western" diets for a month for the sake of science. Instead of consuming a diet of 2,100 to 4,500 calories a day, in which 42 percent of the calories came from fat, 22 percent from high-fiber carbohydrates, 24 percent from refined carbohydrates and 12 percent from protein, they ate only 1,600 to 1,800 calories a day, of which 15 percent came from fat, 65 percent from high-fiber carbohydrates and 20 percent from protein.

At the same time, they cut back their sodium intake by more than 75 percent and reduced their intake of refined carbohydrates to practically zero. As a result, their blood pressure in many cases fell to normal levels. The diet also "reduced the number of patients who would have otherwise received antihypertensive drug therapy" (*Postgraduate Medical Journal,* October, 1983).

When checking your blood pressure, it's wise to have an electrocardiogram (EKG) taken, too. An EKG can show whether or not your heart has ever been damaged by a "silent," or asymptomatic, heart attack. It can also measure left ventricular hypertrophy, a condition which means the heart has become enlarged by the chore of pushing blood through vessels with abnormally high pressure. An EKG can also tell whether or not your heartbeat is irregular.

Testing for these conditions is important because they all increase the risk of stroke. "Your blood pressure might not be very high, it might be only mildly elevated," Dr. Wolf explains. "But if you've got cardiac impairment, your risk of stroke might be as high as someone with very high blood pressure. You'd have to take the problem much more seriously."

Another way to prevent stroke is to prevent or treat diabetes. A history of diabetes or merely the presence of hazardously high levels of sugar in the blood and urine "represents a significant and consistent contributor to stroke risk," according to one study in Holland. Diabetes appeared to more than double the stroke risk (*Stroke,* May/June, 1982).

In explaining why diabetes might promote stroke, researchers at Duke University suggest that excess sugar molecules in the blood somehow interfere with the breakdown of a protein called fibrin. Fibrin is the "glue" that holds blood clots together. If it isn't broken down, unwanted blood clots may form. Each of the clots has the potential to block a blood vessel in the brain and cause a stroke.

Cigarette smokers who are concerned about stroke would

be wise to extinguish their bad habit as soon as possible. Many researchers have downplayed the contribution that smoking makes to the risk of stroke, but others underline its importance. "There was a positive association between the risk of stroke and smoking," say the Framingham researchers, and Finnish men who smoked—in addition to having high blood pressure and high cholesterol levels—were *15.4 times* as likely to suffer a stroke as men without any of those three preconditions.

Indeed, the direct impact of smoking on the cerebral arteries may be highly underestimated. John Meyer, M.D., of the Veterans Administration Medical Center in Houston, believes that smoking reduces the elasticity of the blood vessels and gradually constricts blood flow to the brain. He estimates that smoking multiplies the risk of stroke by a factor of five.

According to Dr. Meyer and his associate Robert L. Rogers, "We've noticed that people who've smoked two or three packs of cigarettes a day for 20 to 30 years very often have strokes." Several years ago, Dr. Meyer began tracking large numbers of smokers and nonsmokers for the purpose of measuring and comparing the amount of blood circulating in their brains. Tests showed that blood flow was lower in the smokers, and that the more cigarettes they smoked, the lower their cerebral blood flow was (*Journal of the American Medical Association,* November 25, 1983).

Simply by measuring blood flow to the brain, Dr. Meyer claims, doctors and patients might be able to predict an impending stroke and possibly to prevent it. "We've found that cerebral blood flow starts to decline about two years before a stroke," Dr. Meyer says. That gives smokers an opportunity to reverse some of the damage that's been done. "We believe there's an increase in blood flow to the brain if the high-risk individual stops smoking," he says. "It may not go back to normal, but it may approach normal."

There's also evidence that magnesium supplements can reduce the risk of stroke. Brain arteries apparently need almost twice as much magnesium as arteries elsewhere in the body and they seem to be more sensitive to fluctuations in the dietary supply of magnesium, one research team has found. If too little magnesium reaches the cells of the arterial walls, the arteries may suddenly contract and trigger a stroke.

That's the theory of researchers Bella Altura, Ph.D., and her husband, Burton Altura, Ph.D., of the Downstate Medical Center in New York. They believe that stroke and magnesium deficiency share many of the same symptoms, such as confusion, hallucinations and depression. That has led them to suggest that magnesium might, in theory, provide a harmless and inexpensive form of insurance against stroke (*Magnesium,* January 3-6, 1982).

"We think it would be beneficial to take a daily supplement of about 250 milligrams of magnesium, in addition to the Recommended Dietary Allowance (RDA) of 350 milligrams a day for men and 300 milligrams for women," Dr. Burton Altura says. "You could be avoiding tremendous vascular consequences."

Vitamin C, the highly versatile nutrient that comes in handy for a remarkably diverse number of ailments, seems to help in stroke prevention, too. British researchers found that people who consume large amounts of fresh fruits and vegetables are less likely to die of stroke. They suspect that the vitamin C in the produce is the active ingredient. They speculate that vitamin C might strengthen the tiny blood vessels in the brain, preventing hemorrhagic strokes, or it may help dissolve dangerous blood clots, preventing clot-induced strokes (*Lancet*, May 28, 1983).

Staying in shape through exercise is another good way to prevent all aspects of circulatory disease, stroke included. In the Netherlands, a team of researchers followed an entire community for several years, monitoring people of all ages for the appearance of virtually all of the stroke risk factors.

The result showed that people who engage in "regular light" as well as "regular heavy" physical activity during their leisure time have only 40 percent of the stroke risk that less athletic people do. "A significant inverse relationship existed between the extent of physical exertion and stroke risk," they say.

There is another form of treatment that is intended to prevent a complete stroke in those people who have already suffered a TIA, or mini-stroke. It is a surgical technique called "carotid thromboendarterectomy."

Very often, TIA survivors have a clot partially blocking

the carotid artery, which is the major supplier of blood to the brain. Such a clot will frequently be located at the point in the neck where the carotid artery branches into two divisions. If so, a vascular surgeon may recommend an endarterectomy. This calls for opening the artery, plucking out the clot and sewing the artery back up again. According to Howard Baron, M.D., a New York City vascular surgeon, endarterectomy can save 85 to 95 percent of all TIA victims from a subsequent and more serious stroke.

The operation isn't for everyone, however. It helps only the 40 to 60 percent of all potential stroke patients whose blockage occurs in the carotid artery. Also, only people younger than 70 are considered strong enough to endure the operation. And, while the operation itself carries a "minimal risk," one of the diagnostic tests used to locate the clot—called an angiogram—can have serious complications. There are, however, other, less hazardous diagnostic techniques.

If there is a silver lining to the stroke problem, it is that the mortality rate from the disease has been steadily declining for the past decade. Although stroke is still the third leading cause of death in this country—of 800,000 or so strokes a year, about 165,000 are fatal—mortality from the disease has fallen by 42 percent since 1972. In the past ten years, it has also been falling faster than ever before.

The reason for this heartening phenomenon is unknown. Some physicians say that the stroke rate started sinking when antihypertension medications became widely prescribed. Others suggest that greater use of vitamin C and less use of salt both play at least a partial role in preventing fatal strokes.

New Approaches
to Better Vision

Most patients would probably think it strange for an eye doctor to ask them how often they exercise, the last time they had a chocolate bar or whether they enjoy their job. After all, what could any of these things possibly have to do with cataracts, glaucoma or even a simple case of dry, itching eyes?

But for Joseph M. Ortiz, M.D., a suburban Philadelphia ophthalmologist, getting answers to questions about diet, exercise, stress and allergies is an important part of the detective work involved in tracking down the cause of an eye problem, or, better yet, stopping one *before* it starts.

That's because Dr. Ortiz believes the most important requirement for healthy eyes is a healthy body. "You can never forget that your eyes are connected to the rest of your body," he says. "They are inseparable."

He's seen the connection again and again—an uncontrollable twitch traced to the stress of a new job and aggravated by too much coffee, a bad case of dry eyes caused by an extremely low-fat diet, computer-induced eyestrain relieved by a new prescription for reading glasses and a no-glare screen. And it goes beyond that.

Your eyes can be hurt by whole-body diseases like high blood pressure, heart disease and diabetes. In fact, looking into the eyes is a good way to see signs of those illnesses. They are the only place in the body where blood vessels can be viewed directly. Clogged, bleeding or scarred vessels in the back part of the eye, called the retina, mean the same problems are occurring elsewhere in the body, Dr. Ortiz says. "They say the eye is the mirror of the soul. Well, it's also a window to look in on the rest of your body." That's why it's no surprise to him that some of his patients who start out treating an eye problem end up with lower blood pressure or extra energy—and a new faith in whole-body healing.

Dr. Ortiz is one of a still-rare breed of preventive ophthalmologists. His training is traditional, with a medical degree from New York Medical College and a residency and research work at Yale and the University of Pennsylvania. He helps supervise a resident-staffed eye clinic at the Hospital of the University of Pennsylvania and admits many of his surgical patients to Wills Eye Hospital or Sheie Eye Institute in Philadelphia.

But his conversion to preventive medicine is wholehearted. After a bout with hepatitis during his freshman year in medical school left him wondering if he would survive to grow old, he gradually changed his diet to emphasize whole grains, vegetables, fruits and some dairy products. Along the way, he monitored the effects of dietary changes with blood tests.

"Those tests really helped me see how cutting out red meat, sugar, coffee, white flour and alcohol improved my blood cholesterol and overall health," he says. And no one can accuse him of not preaching what he practices. He suggests the same menu for his patients.

In fact, his office in Bala Cynwyd, Pennsylvania, with a virtual take-your-pick of holistic medical specialists as neighbors, seems to attract a certain kind of patient—the kind every doctor should be so lucky to have.

"These are people who are actively seeking nutritional care for their eyes," Dr. Ortiz says. "They want a sympathetic, knowledgeable person to give them the information they need. They are well aware of the ways to take care of their bodies, but they have never before had input from an *eye* doctor concerning what they should be doing for their bodies to help their eyes."

Every one of his patients, whether they have an eye problem or not, is encouraged to change his or her diet toward whole grains and fresh produce, to stop smoking and to get plenty of exercise and rest. He recommends vitamin supplements to patients with special problems and older patients.

"If I see previous eye damage—scar tissue or injured blood vessels in the retina—I'll recommend 200 to 400 international units (I.U.) of vitamin E and 50 milligrams of zinc to help maintain the health of the blood vessels and the cells of the retina," he says. "If someone is old, has dentures or doesn't eat much meat, I'll suggest B vitamins, since they may not be getting enough. I think most people get enough vitamin A in their diet, so I reserve that for people with absorption or storage problems—colitis, cirrhosis, or a history of alcoholism. I give them 20,000 to 25,000 I.U. a day."

His surgical patients are "prepped" with 2,000 milligrams of vitamin C, 50 milligrams of zinc and 200 I.U. of vitamin E daily for a week before their operations, and stay on those supplements until they heal. "This reduces inflammation after surgery and cuts up to two weeks off their period of recuperation," Dr. Ortiz says.

For night blindness, the inability of our eyes to adapt to the dark, Dr. Ortiz initially prescribes 50,000 I.U. or more of vitamin A and 75 to 100 milligrams of zinc. After about a month of treatment, he cuts those high doses back. Vitamin A is essential for the health of the cells lining the retina, called rods and cones. And in low-light situations, the chemical impulses of those cells, which send visual images to our brains, require vitamin A to form a light-sensitive pigment known as rhodopsin, or visual purple. Without the pigment, we become virtually blind after dark.

Zinc, Dr. Ortiz says, enhances the eye's ability to use vitamin A. It is important in the conversion of vitamin A to its active form, retinaldehyde. Vitamin E also has an important effect on how much vitamin A is available for use in the eye. It's also been found to be of help as a cataract fighter, Dr. Ortiz believes.

Cataracts, clouding of the eyes' lenses, are an inevitable feature of aging, Dr. Ortiz admits. "Anyone who lives long enough is going to get them." But his own work with some of his patients and laboratory studies with animals have shown that cataract formation in its early stages can be significantly slowed, and in some cases even reversed.

Most researchers believe that a type of cataract found in the aging eye (radiation cataracts) is caused by years of exposure to the sun. "Sunlight absorbed by the lens reacts with an amino acid called tryptophan, breaking it up into particles called free radicals," Dr. Ortiz explains. These destructive, unpaired electrons bind with proteins in the lens, forming the dense pigment that blocks sunlight from the eye and gives it a yellow-brown color.

But laboratory studies have shown that vitamin E and C and the trace mineral selenium block free radicals' destructiveness. Instead of attacking the proteins, free radicals combine with these nutrients and are neutralized.

In patients at an age where cataracts are likely to occur (starting at around 55), Dr. Ortiz suggests 1,500 milligrams of vitamin C and 200 to 400 I.U. of vitamin E. If they have high blood pressure, he recommends that instead of vitamin E they get more selenium—preferably in the form of two or three bulbs of garlic each week. (Selenium supplements should not be taken in amounts more than 200 micrograms daily without a physician's guidance.)

In patients already showing signs of cataracts, Dr. Ortiz pulls out all the stops. Their supplements may include 2,000 milligrams of vitamin C, 400 I.U. of vitamin E, up to 200 micrograms of selenium if needed, and up to 100 milligrams of riboflavin (vitamin B_2). Vitamin E may enhance glutathione, a substance that apparently protects the proteins in the eyes' lenses from free radical damage.

One of Dr. Ortiz's cataract patients is spry 76-year-old Dr. Ibraham Marker. This man lost the use of one eye several years earlier when blood vessels in his retina burst. When he realized cataracts were destroying his remaining vision, he was determined to find a doctor who would help him without requiring surgery. After three months of Dr. Ortiz's eye regimen, Dr. Marker's eyesight had improved dramatically. With glasses, visual acuity in his "good" eye had improved from 20/100 to 20/60. Even his retina-damaged eye showed an improvement— from 20/400 to 20/200.

"This man is a remarkable example of how nutritional supplements can work to improve the health of the retina," Dr. Ortiz says. "You have to use total body care to help your eyes. This man is in good health. He eats carefully, is very active and does a lot of walking. I think the reason supplements helped him so much is that he takes such good care of himself. Eventually he may need cataract surgery, but at this time both he and I are satisfied with his improved vision."

Dr. Ortiz's diabetic patients, because they are especially prone to cataracts and retinal damage, receive additional advice and supplements.

"I tell them to bring their blood glucose level down to 140, not by increasing their medication but by changing their diet. I also recommend 200 to 400 micrograms of chromium a day. Chromium makes insulin work more efficiently in the body and so helps lower blood sugar levels." A too-high blood sugar level can damage blood vessels in the retina, creating a condition called diabetic retinopathy, which eventually leads to blindness.

To further protect the eyes' blood source, Dr. Ortiz recommends a supplement of eicosapentanoic acid (EPA, a substance in fish oil that helps lower blood cholesterol and triglyceride levels and prevents clumping of blood platelets). This helps to lessen the fatty buildup, clotting and hemorrhaging that can destroy the retina.

In some cases, he also recommends bioflavonoids, nutrients found in the white peel of citrus fruits. Bioflavonoids keep capillary walls strong, helping to prevent leakage from blood vessels. Some bioflavonoids may also work to inhibit an enzyme, aldose reductase, that promotes some kinds of cataracts.

Glaucoma, a dangerous buildup of fluid in the eye that can permanently damage the retina, is another condition that can respond to nutritional therapy, though it usually first requires traditional medical treatment.

"I never start off using vitamins to treat glaucoma," Dr. Ortiz says. "The main thing is to get the pressure down as quickly as possible, using eye drops sometimes supplemented by laser surgery to 'drill' pinpoint holes in the eye through which the fluid can drain."

Then, if the pressure has to be brought down a little further, Dr. Ortiz will suggest vitamin C. This treatment is effective only in large doses. "The vitamin C acts as an osmotic agent," he explains. "It draws fluid away from the eye."

In myopia, or nearsightedness, glasses can cause the tiny muscles that focus the eyes' lenses to become very strong, thereby stretching the outer layer of the eyes, Dr. Ortiz explains. Removing the glasses makes the muscles work less and the eye stretching is decreased. This may stabilize the myopia. It also trains your brain to interpret visual messages even though they're not clearly in focus.

"My glasses had gotten thicker and thicker and I always thought the end result of it would be that I would go blind or something," says Myrna Miller, one of Dr. Ortiz's patients. "It's really heartening when you can put that in reverse and keep it there."

Mrs. Miller had the time and patience to go without her glasses. Not everyone can do that or have the results Mrs. Miller had, but they still can be active participants in their eye care, Dr. Ortiz says.

Good Stuff for a Stuffy Head

A stuffed-up nose isn't just unpleasant. It's unhealthy. Chronic stuffiness can indicate physical obstructions, such as a deviated septum or nasal polyps, or chronic irritations like allergies. It can make you work harder to get the air you need and cause sleeping problems. Some doctors believe it may even be a sign of underlying psychological problems.

If your stuffy nose is chronic, you should be checked for structural defects, says Stanley Farb, M.D., author of *The Ear, Nose and Throat Book: A Doctor's Guide to Better Health Care* (Prentice-Hall). "But inhalant allergies are more commonly a cause, and most people know if that's their problem," Dr. Farb says. "If your stuffiness happens only during a certain time of year, or when you mow the lawn or smell mothballs, you can pretty much pinpoint the cause." Avoiding that irritant or simply using an antihistamine during contact may be all you need to do, Dr. Farb says.

If your allergy symptoms are long-lasting and severe, tests and desensitizing shots may be your choice. An air conditioner, air filters on your heating system or electrostatic precipitators, especially in your bedroom, may also help, Dr. Farb says. You can often rent these appliances before you make a purchase to see if they work for you.

If allergy tests prove negative or shots don't help, suspect food or chemical problems. "You can be just as blocked up by these as by pollen," says Marshall Mandell, M.D., author of the *Five-Day Allergy Relief System* (Thomas Crowell) and medical director of the Alan Mandell Center for Bio-Ecologic Diseases, Norwalk, Connecticut. "Most allergists give this a fancy name—like vasomotor rhinitis or rhinosinusitis—but they don't do anything about it. I think that's a cop-out."

Find a doctor in this field or try playing detective yourself, keeping a diary of everything you eat, your activities and exposures to connect symptoms with exposure to certain foods or chemicals.

Some of the more common foods that can cause nasal allergies are milk (especially in children), coffee (especially in adults), wheat, eggs, beef, pork, sugar, yeast, corn and tomatoes.

Any of the other foods that you eat two or three times a week might also play an important role in this condition.

Perhaps the easiest way to find out if a food is causing your stuffy nose is to eliminate it from your diet for a week to see if your symptoms disappear. Then, eat it again and see if they return. Keep in mind that it's possible to be allergic to 10 or 15 foods and taking one of them out of your diet may not eliminate your symptoms. If, for one week, however, you follow a simple diet of foods not usually eaten (and do not use pepper, ketchup, mustard, sugar or other spices or flavorings), Dr. Mandell feels you may eliminate just about all the offenders and clear your symptoms.

Don't forget, too, that many environmental chemicals, such as chlorinated water, natural gas and cigarette smoke, may be irritants for some people.

If your symptoms don't seem to fit any of these categories, check for blood-pressure medicines that contain reserpine, as well as birth control pills, replacement estrogen, an under-active thyroid gland, or aspirin sensitivity. You may need the assistance of your doctor in this matter.

Try a humidifier or vaporizer if the mucus in your nose is thick or your nose seems dry. "These work especially well for colds during the winter months," Dr. Farb says. They may actually aggravate some allergies, though, by producing a moist environment that promotes the growth of molds.

For temporary relief, try hot drinks, which speed up the flow of mucus through the nose. Sip chicken soup or teas made with natural decongestants like fenugreek, anise or sage. Hot and spicy foods also thin out mucus. So do garlic and onions. Your breath might be impossible, but at least you'll be able to breathe for a while.

Exercise often temporarily unblocks a stuffy nose. It produces direct nervous stimulation to the nose and changes in blood chemistry—more adrenaline, for instance—which helps shrink and dry up nasal tissues.

Using salt water to "wash" your nose is an old remedy suggested by both traditional and alternative doctors. Salt water thins out mucus, making it easier for the body to expel. It also rinses dust and pollen from the nose. "Nasal douching has been around for a long time, and we find it very effective in helping to relieve stuffiness and infection," says Lawrence Cohen, M.D., coordinator of the Himalayan Institute's Dana Research Laboratory, Honesdale, Pennsylvania. He uses an Eastern contraption called a neti pot, filled with four ounces of lukewarm water and ⅛ to ¼ teaspoon of kosher salt, which contains no iodine or silicates. Other doctors suggest using a nose dropper.

Shoring up your body's defenses with the vitamins and minerals shown to help allergies and colds might be your best all-around bet.

"To make a person healthier with good nutrition is a basic concept," Dr. Mandell says. "It only stands to reason that appropriate nutritional supplementation can also make people more resistant to allergies, but this is something most allergists haven't the faintest notion about."

His "antipollutant, antioxidant" program, as he puts it, includes vitamins C, E, A and B complex, plus bioflavonoids and selenium, zinc and other minerals.

Vitamin C gives the immune system a boost, It also acts as a natural antihistamine, helping to reduce inflammation of the mucous membranes, Dr. Mandell says. "A number of allergy patients tell me their intake of vitamin C determines whether their allergies will be mild or severe." His patients take five grams or more a day.

Vitamins E, A and C also help maintain the integrity of the cells at the forefront of the air pollution assault. Vitamin E is considered the best antioxidant of all. Some people report obtaining allergy or sinus relief by dripping the contents of a vitamin E capsule into their nose. Some all-natural nasal sprays include vitamin E in their formula.

Fasting: What Can It Really Do for You?

After he had suffered for six years with colitis, gone through more than 40 different drugs and an operation to remove gangrenous hemorrhoids, Jack Goldstein, D.P.M., wasn't looking for any more trouble. But it came one day when his doctor said the time had come for surgery.

But the 34-year-old Michigan podiatrist decided on something to which his doctor, and most others, would strongly object. He stopped eating.

Dr. Goldstein actually went on a supervised fast at a New York health retreat specializing in "the ultimate diet." The only thing that passed through his lips was spring water—no medicines, no vitamins, not even a little toothpaste paté on the side.

Six weeks later and 40 pounds lighter, Dr. Goldstein felt weak but "physically reborn," as he puts it. No, his colitis wasn't completely cured. But it was better than it had been in a long time, and without drugs. It would take years of careful eating and more periodic fasts to keep his problem under control. But Dr. Goldstein believes the fast gave his body the rest it needed to focus all its energy on healing.

That's something most of today's medical experts scoff at. They think fasting is useless, and that it can be deadly. Dr. Goldstein's own physician decided the improvement was psychological. And a biologist from Pennsylvania, who notes that fasting slows the growth of intestinal cells, says going without food should actually have interfered with healing and aggravated the disease.

Their conclusions, Dr. Goldstein says, "just show how little most doctors really know about fasting, and how little they care to learn." But even he admits the dangers of what was for him a last resort. "Just because it helped me doesn't mean everybody should or can do it safely. I don't think anyone should fast more than a day or two without proper supervision."

What is fasting? Is it safe? Are there any accepted medical reasons for doing it? The answers seem to depend on whom you ask. And there are many questions yet to be answered when it comes to any kind of scientific basis for fasting's reported benefits.

To fast means to abstain. "Fasting is a voluntary abstinence from any food or liquid that contains calories," says Allan Cott, M.D., a New York City orthomolecular psychiatrist who has used fasting to help schizophrenics. Dr. Cott is the author of *Fasting: The Ultimate Diet* (Bantam Books).

The longest reported fasts were by two patients treated at a hospital in Scotland, according to Nevin Scrimshaw, M.D., Ph.D., of the Massachusetts Institute of Technology. One was a 30-year-old woman who ate no food for 236 days and reduced from 281 to 184 pounds. The other, a 54-year-old woman, went 249 days and dropped from 282 to 208 pounds. Neither woman showed any significant side effects that could be attributed to lack of food, doctors noted.

There have been several deaths reported among fasting obese patients, Dr. Scrimshaw says, but in all but one case the deaths apparently were due to preexisting medical problems that had been aggravated by the weight problem, not fasting. The one exception was a 20-year-old English woman who in 30 weeks of total fasting went from 260 to 132 pounds.

On the seventh day after she had resumed eating, her heartbeat became irregular. Two days later she died. An autopsy revealed she had burned up half of the muscle tissue in her body, including part of her heart.

But a properly supervised fast would end long before such damage could occur. Such a fast could even have therapeutic value, slowing the gastrointestinal reflex and resting the body.

"You know that saying, 'Feed a cold, starve a fever'? Well, we believe that if you feed a cold, you will *have* to starve a fever," says James Lennon, assistant executive director of the Natural Hygiene Society of Tampa, Florida, an organization that advocates fasting as part of a total health program. "When you are ill, you're going to have a hard time digesting food, and that could make you even sicker. Animals actually have more sense when it comes to this. They know enough to stop eating until they feel better."

Skipping a few meals when you're feverish or nauseated is a lot different, though, from fasting for days or weeks to treat ailments like arthritis or colitis, says George Blackburn, M.D., Ph.D., a Harvard Medical School professor of surgery who has studied some of the physical effects of fasting.

"There are no known therapeutic reasons for a total fast, not even weight loss, because the dramatic change in body metabolism it creates could cause organ failure and disease, and the composition of the weight loss would be an unacceptable amount of body fluid and tissue protein from muscles and organs," Dr. Blackburn says.

Most of the benefits seen in fasting come from food reduction and weight loss, and could be produced much more safely with a prudent diet, he says. "It's true that eating, particularly overeating, creates major metabolic stress on the body. It can produce a harmful excess of adrenaline and insulin. Cutting down does lessen hormone stimulation and allows the body to feel better." Could it even help the body to live longer?

Researchers at the Gerontology Research Center in Baltimore found that rats fed every other day lived 63 weeks longer than their cage mates, who were allowed to eat all they wanted. They also remained more active later in life.

Dr. Blackburn agrees. "Fasting for one day isn't going to hurt you, and if these animal studies are an indication, it may be of some benefit. It's a longer fast that concerns me."

Fasting, like any diet where you eat fewer calories than you burn, forces your body to consume its own tissues to stay alive, says James Naughton, M.D., a professor of medicine at the University of California at San Francisco, who has a special interest in fasting.

Normally after a meal, the body uses the glucose from the meal to provide energy to the brain and other organs. It also stores some glucose in the liver and muscles.

When you haven't eaten for 12 hours or so, the body begins to use the glucose stored in the liver. That supply, though, lasts less than a day.

The muscles then begin to break down their own protein for energy, and release amino acids, which are converted to glucose. This is the major source of energy for the brain and nervous system from the second to about the fourteenth day of a fast, and with it goes a large loss of salt, water and protein. (In fact, up to half the weight lost early in a fast is water that is quickly regained when eating resumes, Dr. Blackburn says.)

But as the fast and the breakdown of tissues continues, body chemistry changes. More and more fat goes to the liver, where it is broken down into compounds called ketones. After about three or four days of fasting, the body starts producing ketones for energy. The body slowly burns more and more ketones and less glucose, so that by about the twenty-first day of the fast, it's burning 90 percent fat and 10 percent protein. It continues at this ratio until it uses up its store of fat. Then, the body makes a final fatal dip into its protein supplies in the muscles and organs. Weakened chest muscles and the inability to clear secretions from the lungs make pneumonia the leading cause of fasting deaths. Fatal heart arrhythmia may also occur.

There are risks at the beginning of a fast, too, Dr. Blackburn contends. "Protein and mineral losses are front-ended. They start after 24 hours and continue for several weeks. Short fasts of 3 days, a week, 20 days, tear the guts out of the body tissue and could lead to a heart attack or stroke."

Those risks exist for someone with heart disease, artery blockage or poor nutritional status, says Dr. Naughton. "But a healthy person seems to be able to tolerate protein and mineral losses during that time without much difficulty."

Both agree kidney stones and gout can be a problem for some fasters, too.

But some good things can also happen while you're fasting. Blood sugar and insulin levels drop, says Dr. Naughton. While they rise again when eating is resumed, insulin levels don't always go as high as they were before the fast, possibly because glucose-starved cells have become more sensitive to insulin. But you could get these same effects dieting off excess pounds, Dr. Naughton says.

During a fast your blood pressure also drops, sometimes so much that you feel faint. This is caused by an initial large loss of water and sodium. But blood pressure quickly rises when the fast is ended, and any permanent lowering is the result of weight loss.

Hunger, the constant companion of many other diets, decreases by the third or fourth day of a fast. And the mental lethargy, apathy and irritability seen during periods of semi-starvation are less prominent in total fasting, Dr. Naughton says. In fact, many fasters report a sense of well-being, euphoria and clearheadedness.

Some of these effects may be psychological, as voluntary

fasters report them more often than forced fasters, Dr. Naughton says. But others may be the result of altered brain chemistry.

Both Russian and British researchers have reported that fasting raised the level of serotonin, a neurotransmitter that plays a role in mood and the ability to perceive pleasure, Dr. Cott says.

And recently, scientists at the University of Athens discovered that food deprivation blocks the brain's uptake of dopamine, another neurotransmitter. That finding was particularly interesting to Dr. Cott, because the medications used to treat schizophrenia do the same thing, he says.

"I've fasted about 300 chronically ill schizophrenics, people who would have ended up in the back wards of mental hospitals," he says. After about 25 to 32 days without food, 65 percent had improved enough to return to some degree of functioning and leave the hospital. Those who stayed on a vegetarian diet after the fast were least likely to relapse, he says.

But fasting's not for everyone, even its advocates agree. And it shouldn't be for *anyone* without an understanding of its risks, and competent medical supervision.

Infection Protection for Senior Citizens

A hundred years ago, scientists discovered an interesting phenomenon. As people grew older, their organ weights changed. Lungs, liver and brain weigh slightly less in an 80-year-old than they do in a 20-year-old. And the thymus actually shrinks to a mere fraction of its original size. It was only about 20 years ago that this phenomenon went from interesting to significant. That was when scientists learned the function of the thymus, a flat, pinkish-gray, two-lobed gland that nestles behind the sternum and lungs high in the chest. Put simply, the thymus distributes and nourishes (with its hormones) white blood cells, called lymphocytes, that act as the body's army against disease.

The thymus appears to be the command headquarters for

an army of cells known as T lymphocytes, which, when they meet a foreign invader like a virus or cancer cell, can be stimulated to divide into larger, active cells that react with the invader and kill it. At the same time, the T cells seem to stimulate other parts of the immune system into action: the macrophages, PacMan-like scavengers that literally gobble up the enemy, known as antigens, and B cells, which the T cells encourage to produce antibodies against the antigen.

If your immune system is working at its optimum, right now the T cells in your body could be leading a battle against cancer or infection without your even knowing it.

But in aging, the thymus, at its maximum when we are teenagers, shrinks markedly, leaving us with less of the nourishing thymic hormones and fewer young T cells to replenish our aged army. The aged T cells decline in their ability to reproduce and to stimulate the B cells to produce antibodies. "As a unifying concept, what is happening is that the control of the immune system begins to decline with age," says William Adler, M.D., chief of the clinical immunology section, Gerontology Research Center, National Institute on Aging, Baltimore.

This shrinking of the thymus and resultant decline in T-cell function is believed to be largely responsible for the increasing illness and death rates among the elderly, particularly for cancer and infection, which until now have been considered simply part of the aging process.

Fortunately, that assumption has been called into question. "There is at least a distinct possibility that some illness and abnormalities we are seeing in the immune response in the elderly may not be a part of the normal aging process, that there are environmental factors, particularly diet, that may have a causal role to play," says Ranjit Kumar Chandra, M.D., of the Health Sciences Center, Memorial University of Newfoundland.

In 1984 Dr. Chandra organized an international conference on nutrition, immunity and illness in the elderly, drawing scientists from North America, Europe, Scandinavia and even Japan to St. Johns, Newfoundland, to discuss the possibilities for intervening in the process that leaves the elderly so vulnerable to disease.

One prime area of research involves the thymic hormones. Researcher William Ershler, M.D., of the University of Vermont School of Medicine, has studied the effects of the thymic hormone thymosin on human lymphocytes in the test tube. When he added a dose of thymosin to test tubes containing white blood cells of aged subjects who had received shots for tetanus and influenza, the elderly cells were stimulated to produce a normal amount of antibodies, something they were unable to do before. Next, Dr. Ershler says he hopes to test thymosin outside the test tube, in elderly people inoculated against flu. But it may be some time before thymosin becomes the treatment of choice for the aging immune system. There may be a more immediate, self-administered treatment, says the researcher. "You may consider taking zinc," he advises, "since some researchers in immunology and aging have shown a clear benefit in the immune system, experimentally, with zinc."

The reason? The thymus is chock-full of zinc, which is essential to both protein synthesis and cell division. Since the efficient working of the immune system depends on the rapid proliferation of cells, it's not surprising that the prescription calls for zinc.

And zinc was the answer to a paradox that confronted Robert Good, M.D., Ph.D., head of the cancer research program at the Oklahoma Medical Research Foundation. In his fieldwork among malnourished children, he and his colleagues noted that malnutrition was accompanied by a profound decline in immunity. Children whose calories and protein were restricted were far more susceptible to disease and infection. Yet, in well-known laboratory studies, restriction of protein and calories in animals prolonged their lives.

What Dr. Good discovered was that it was not the protein or calorie deprivation that caused the drop in immunological function, but the lack of zinc. And other researchers have found that it is possible to correct the immunological malfunction just by giving the children zinc, before correcting anything else, says Dr. Good.

Dr. Chandra, who has also done extensive field research on immunodeficiency among malnourished children, tested the immune response in a group of elderly whose diets were supplemented with zinc for six weeks.

He gave them a skin test—injecting a variety of antigens largely derived from bacteria and molds into the superficial layers of their skin. In a normal, healthy person, at least one of the spots should show a swollen, inflamed reaction in about two days, meaning the lymphocytes are proliferating and the immune system has swung into action. It is not unusual for many elderly people to show no reaction to the skin test, indicating their immune systems are not mobilized to fight a threatening disease. Not surprisingly, this lack of reaction is a fairly accurate predictor of death. "Those elderly individuals who are found to be anergic (nonreactive) often die in the next three to five years," says Dr. Chandra.

But zinc may be able to change those odds. In Dr. Chandra's zinc-supplemented group, at least half increased their number of responses to the skin test, indicating there was some new life in their immune systems.

The very latest research strengthens the case for zinc. A group of scientists in Italy has discovered that at least one of the thymic hormones, called FTS, is not so much affected by the shrinking of the thymus as it is by the kind of marginal zinc deficiencies so prevalent among the elderly.

They noticed that children with Down's syndrome and elderly people had a similar lack of active circulating FTS and zinc. The finding intrigued them because Down's syndrome children "show at an early age normal subjective factors of aging, such as autoimmunity, an increase in leukemia, the graying of hair and cataracts," says researcher Claudio Franceschi, M.D., professor of immunology at the University of Padua, Italy.

That led him to consider the possibility that the shrinking thymus was taking the blame for a failure of the FTS hormone. "The glands work," says the researcher, "but produce inactive molecules." Blood samples taken from the two groups turned up a substance that was capable of inhibiting the activity of FTS in the test tube. When zinc was added to the culture, it induced concentrations of FTS comparable to those of normal, healthy young people.

What Dr. Franceschi and his colleagues believe is that FTS is biologically bound to zinc, and needs it to be active and effective. Dr. Franceschi speculates that this inhibitory factor found in the blood samples was FTS hormone not bound to zinc. "When we added zinc, the hormone was able to bind itself to the zinc molecules to become active," he says.

But the clinical results speak more than the test-tube studies. When the Down's syndrome children were given relatively small amounts of zinc as a dietary supplement (one milligram per kilogram [2.2 pounds] of body weight), the results were remarkable. "Though it's difficult to measure," says Dr. Franceschi, "the children had less infections and lost fewer days at school. We think this is directly related to the zinc."

But zinc isn't the only nutrient under current investigation. Several researchers are probing the effects of vitamin E on the aging immune system. One of them is Simin Meydani, a scientist with a unique pedigree—she is a veterinarian with a Ph.D. in human nutrition. Dr. Meydani, a senior research associate at Brandeis University and a consultant at the USDA Human Nutrition Center at Tufts University in Boston, tested vitamin E on immune responsiveness in aged mice.

"We supplemented aged mice with vitamin E and compared the effects by measuring different parameters of immune response," she explains. The supplemented mice showed an improvement in their responses to skin tests similar to those given by Dr. Chandra to his elderly human subjects. And in the test tube, lymphocyte proliferation was significantly improved by vitamin E supplementation.

A group of scientists in Belgium tested the effects of another potential immunity booster, vitamin C, in a group of healthy volunteers over 70. One group was treated for a month with intramuscular injections of 500 milligrams of vitamin C—many times the recommended daily allowance—while the other group was treated with a placebo injection of saline solution.

The group that received the vitamin C had better skin-test responses to tuberculine antigens and, in the test tube, their lymphocytes were more active when exposed to a stimulatory substance.

One of the reasons for the results may be the role vitamin C plays in helping thymic hormones in their job of changing immature, inactive T lymphocytes into cells ready to battle disease, the researchers suggest (*Gerontology,* vol. 29, no. 5, 1983).

Soak Away Your Aches and Pains

Few of those familiar with the peculiar antics of Blanche DuBois would deny the woman was a bit of an oddball. In fact, her brother-in-law considered her downright loony—especially when he had to put up with her irritating habit of steaming up the house on 100-degree evenings with the vapors coming from the bathroom as she soaked in a hot bath.

But Blanche was insistent: "Oh, I feel so good after my long, hot bath, I feel so good and cool and—rested."

While such a comment only stoked the already burning suspicions about the mental state of the Tennessee Williams character, Blanche may not have been as daft as others in *A Streetcar Named Desire* made her out to be—at least where her penchant for hot soaks on hot nights was concerned.

"It only makes sense that a hot soak could help you cool off, even on a summer night," says D.L. Moore, M.D., medical director at Living Springs Retreat in Putnam Valley, New York. Why? Because a hot-water bath—from about 102° to 110°F—is one of the best ways to clear away the fats and salts that accumulate on the skin, especially during hot weather. And, as hot water caresses the skin, the veins dilate, allowing the heat to hasten its escape outside the body. The result? You feel good, you feel cool—just like Blanche said.

"It's the body's way of naturally trying to maintain temperature equilibrium," agrees Richard R. Mautz, a registered physical therapist from the Weimar (California) Institute. "If you give it heat, it reacts by cooling down; if you give it cool water, it'll want to warm up."

"Water is a very simple solution to many everyday ills, yet people too often think of turning to drugs instead," says Dr. Moore. "They don't even think of turning to water. Yet water has been used successfully in the treatment of more diseases than any other remedy." And water has one up on drugs in other ways, too. It's inexpensive, in abundant supply and natural.

So, then, what are the medicinal qualities of water that make it such a divine healer? For one, water has the enormous capacity to cause action and reaction in the three most important systems of the body: the nervous system (including the brain, spinal cord and nerves), the heart and circulatory system and the skin. It also stimulates the metabolism.

For example, hot water increases circulation in any part of the body it may touch. It can act as a counterirritant—the soothing feeling of hot water moving over the spine can transcend the feeling of ache and pain. And, depending on the temperature and length of soaking, hot water can either perk you up or calm you down. Just how you're going to get these great benefits, of course, depends a lot on the method of hot soak you use. But before we get into the glorious options, a few words of caution.

All the experts we talked to emphasize that most hot soaks should be followed by a cold splash. The reason is that hot water—say, anything above 104°F—slows the movement of oxygen to the brain. And that you don't want. However, a quick cool-down with cold water—30 seconds will do just fine—starts to return oxygen flow to normal. Also, anyone with heart disease, high blood pressure or diabetes is best off staying away from any extreme temperature dunks without asking their doctor first.

Now for the best of hot-water soaks, starting with Blanche's favorite.

"There is probably nothing in the world better for relaxing the muscles than a hot bath," says Dr. Moore. "Whether muscle tightness is from disease, fatigue or strain, people often find great relief soaking in a hot tub."

By hot we mean anything from around 100° to 110°F, with 102° to 104°F the ideal. Anything too hot—particularly above 110°F—is not recommended, says Dr. Moore. "Prolonged use (30 minutes or more) of water that is too hot will stimulate the heart and be exhausting."

The real value of a hot-water soak is the relief it can bring to the millions suffering from that scourge of aging—arthritis. "Gently moving the joints while soaking in a hot tub can help improve mobility in patients with arthritis," says Carole Lewis, Ph.D., codirector of Physical Therapy Services of Washington, D.C., Inc., and an adjunct assistant professor at the University of Pittsburgh. "For these people, just sitting in the tub and relaxing is not enough. They should move. Simple and gentle stretches in water can help improve range of motion."

A hot-water soak is ideal for arthritics because body weight is lighter in water, making exercises all that much easier. In fact, those with arthritis find that what they can't do *out* of water they can do *in* water.

If your arthritis makes it difficult for you to get into a tub, here's a simple technique recommended in *Natural Relief for Arthritis,* by Carol Keough (Rodale Press, 1983). Step into the tub with your back to the faucets, get down on your hands and knees and slowly slide into a sitting position. You can pivot one foot against the side to steady yourself. To get out, first drain the tub, then reverse the procedure.

Frederick R. Rossiter, M.D., author of *Water for Healing and Health,* says a hot-water bath can give relief from painful menstruation. Itching, too, can be relieved with a hot bath, says yet another expert.

Now lower the temperature a tad, to about 98°F or so (our experts call this a *warm* bath), and you have the ideal climate for soothing an array of other ills, with insomnia at the head of the list.

"There is nothing in the world better for insomnia than a warm bath," Dr. Moore states flatly. "It beats any tranquilizer, and it's not addictive." He suggests 15 minutes in a warm tub right before crawling under the covers as one of the best cures for sleeplessness.

Lower the temperature a tad more, to between 92° and 97°F, and you'll have what is called a *neutral* bath. What can a neutral bath do that a hot one can't? For one thing, a neutral bath has a more sedative and soporific effect than a hot bath. It relaxes the blood vessels of the skin. It also soothes nerve endings, helping to calm you down when you're feeling nervous. In fact, before the advent of tranquilizing drugs, neutral baths were used with great success in calming agitated mental patients.

And the benefits go on. Neutral baths can help ease the pain of skin burns, increase activity in the kidneys, reduce skin irritation caused by Bright's disease and hives and help reduce a fever.

Anything a hot bath can do a hot tub can do better. "The agitation of the hot water jets against the skin can help relieve sore muscles and induce relaxation," says Dr. Moore. Better yet is the whirlpool, the stainless steel or ceramic version of the hot tub usually found in hospitals and spas. A whirlpool has stronger action than a hot tub, which only enhances the massaging effect.

Nevertheless, it's only prudent to step into a hot tub with caution. Although it may seem like the social thing to do, drinking alcoholic beverages should be avoided. Death by drowning has been blamed more than once on hot-tub happy hours. Also, hot-tub water should not be too hot; it could cause the bather to pass out. Even though hot tubs are made to withstand much higher temperatures, a safe range is about the same as you'd want your hot bath—about 104°F.

Have a headache? Then go soak your feet. It's one of the most valuable methods found for getting rid of a head-ache, experts say. While it may sound a little like getting to the attic through the cellar door, in theory it really does make a lot of sense. "It's both a reflex and a supply-and-demand reaction," says Mautz, who uses the method on his patients all the time.

"Some headaches are caused by too much blood in the head, causing congestion of the blood vessels," he explains.

"If you soak your feet in hot water, the vessels in the feet dilate, drawing more blood to the feet. Since you only have so much blood in the body, the blood that's going to the feet must come at the expense of other parts of the body, namely the head, where the buildup is."

But hot foot baths are more than just good for the head. If you feel chilled on a cold winter day, a hot foot bath will help you get warm. (If the feet are warm, you know, you'll be warm, too.) And, it's also great for the obvious—sore, tired feet.

To take a hot foot bath, use a small basin or bucket just big enough to hold your feet. Water should be above the ankles, at a temperature of about 110°F. It can last anywhere from 5 to 20 minutes.

At the Weimar Institute, where patients are coached to a healthier lifestyle through a 25-day nondrug treatment program, steam baths are a big part of daily therapy. And their most successful use is in helping people to give up smoking.

Because of their intense heat (up to 122°F), steam baths bring on considerable perspiration. "The sweating helps free the body of nicotine. The heat also stimulates nerve endings, which may replace the stimulating effects of nicotine and thus reduce the physiological need for cigarettes," says Mautz. "Of course the steam bath can't help the mental addiction."

Mautz says Weimar clinicians also have noted a reduction in blood pressure after a steam bath. "It only lasts for three or four hours, but it is noticeable," he says. And, a steam bath is great for relieving muscle spasms.

"We get a lot of hikers here and they say the steam bath is the best thing for getting the kinks out after a long day on the trail," says Mautz.

Sounds nice, doesn't it? But what if you want to *prevent* aches and pains? What if you want to ward off colds and feel good, robust and clearheaded? What's the best water treatment for keeping away disease and keeping the body shipshape? The shower, all our experts agree—the *hot-and-cold* shower.

Start with the hot—as hot as you can stand it. Let the hot water glide over your body, twisting so you can feel its effects on different body parts. (It's not necessary to move your feet; that could cause a fall.) Enjoy the hot water for about three minutes. Then turn the water to cold—as cold as you can stand it—but this time for only 15 to 30 seconds. Repeat three to five times, always ending with cold.

"There is no better protection against colds than this hot-and-cold jet spray, particularly when begun early in life and practiced consistently," says Dr. Rossiter. "This is due to establishing tone in the circulation and resistance in the skin and mucous membranes."

Food and Nutrition Developments

Should You Drink to Your Health?

Arthur Klatsky, M.D., Gary D. Friedman, M.D., and their colleagues at Kaiser-Permanente Medical Center, Oakland, just didn't know what to make of their findings ten years ago. And today they still view them with some puzzlement.

In 1974 Dr. Klatsky, head of cardiology at the center, was asked to conduct a study to look for predictors of heart attacks. Using a computer, he was to review thousands of medical exams, comparing the health histories of people who had gone on to have heart attacks with those who hadn't. Already known predictors—high cholesterol, high blood pressure, diabetes, smoking, overweight—were to be controlled so they would not affect the results. Dr. Klatsky was to look for new, unknown risk factors. Large-scale, open-ended statistical studies like these are called "fishing expeditions," so perhaps it's only fitting that Dr. Klatsky should open up a can of worms.

He did find a number of new predictors. But one in particular stood out. People who had reported in their medical history that they drank no alcohol went on to have about a third more heart attacks and 20 percent more sudden, fatal heart attacks, than those who said they were light to moderate drinkers. ("Light to moderate drinkers" had two or fewer drinks a day. One drink is considered 1½ ounces of 80-proof whiskey, 5 ounces of wine or one 12-ounce bottle of beer.)

"We were afraid of this finding, in a sense," Dr. Klatsky says. "We challenged it in every way we could think of in that first report. We really didn't know what to make of it because it had never been found before."

But since then a number of other studies have produced similar findings in population groups throughout the United States and around the world. In Chicago, Florida, Scotland, Yugoslavia and Israel, the conclusions have been the same— moderate drinkers seem to be healthier than teetotalers. Even the well-known Framingham study, a 24-year-long medical analysis of the residents of a Massachusetts town, was analyzed recently for links between alcohol intake and disease. A slightly lower death rate for all diseases, not just heart disease, was found in people drinking from 1 to 9 ounces of alcohol a month. (That ranges from one 1½-ounce shot of whiskey every 15 days to a shot every other day, or from 2 to 20 bottles of beer a month.)

And that analysis found that even heavier drinkers (who consumed four shots, four glasses of wine or four cans of beer a day) died in no greater numbers than nondrinkers.

In another computer scan of Kaiser-Permanente medical records, Dr. Klatsky compared total deaths, not just deaths from heart attacks, with alcohol intake. He found that people having two or fewer drinks a day still fared best. Teetotalers and those downing three to five drinks a day had the same death rate, which was 50 percent higher than that of moderate drinkers. Moderate drinkers also spent less time in the hospital than either teetotalers or heavier drinkers.

An analysis of all of these studies was done by Thomas Turner, M.D., former dean of the Johns Hopkins Medical School, Baltimore, and now president of the Alcoholic Beverage Medical Research Foundation at Johns Hopkins. "In every one, the rates for cardiovascular deaths and coronary heart disease deaths were lower for moderate drinkers than for either the low- or high-intake groups," he says.

Dr. Turner's analysis also showed a kind of "ceiling" for alcohol intake, an average amount above which deaths tended to increase. "The total death rate did not change significantly until alcohol intake reached six drinks per day," he says. "At that point, total mortality rates for all causes of death were elevated" (*Johns Hopkins Medical Journal,* February, 1981).

So what are we to think of all this? Does it mean a few

drinks a day—possibly even up to six—could actually "preserve" our health, or at least not hurt us?

The numbers from these population studies would seem to indicate yes, but simply too many unanswered questions remain to say it's okay for a doctor to prescribe a few swigs or for a patient to self-administer in the hope of doing himself some good, Dr. Klatsky and Dr. Turner say. Both liver and brain damage could occur in sensitive individuals. And they both personally recommend lower "do not exceed" levels.

"A simplistic view of alcohol as being good or bad for your heart is not appropriate," Dr. Klatsky says. "I don't think drinking should be a mainstay of heart attack prevention. Some people simply want to find some justification to drink heavily, and there's no doubt of the serious harm that can do."

Let's take a look at the arguments pro and con for moderate drinking. First, the statistics.

"Keep in mind that although every one of these studies shows a correlation between moderate alcohol drinking and improved health, a correlation doesn't necessarily mean cause and effect," Dr. Turner says. In other words, moderate drinkers may not necessarily be healthier because they drink.

Could other differences account for the discrepancies? Could moderate drinkers be more sociable or easygoing than their nonimbibing friends, traits that would likely contribute to overall health? Or could teetotalers be physically weaker somehow? Might they avoid drinking because of health problems?

"Those are good questions," Dr. Klatsky says. "One of the basic problems remaining is whether nondrinkers are different from drinkers in ways other than that they don't drink." Most studies *do* separate former heavy drinkers from the nondrinking group. These people do have a higher death rate than lifetime abstainers.

Another problem is that these are statistical analyses, not laboratory studies, says Burton Altura, Ph.D., a physiology professor at the State University of New York's Downstate Medical Center, Brooklyn.

"There is no scientific evidence either in controlled human studies or animal studies which shows that daily low ingestion of alcohol is beneficial to the cardiovascular system," Dr. Altura says.

And he's concerned that even if alcohol does benefit the heart, it could damage the brain or liver in sensitive people. True, Dr. Klatsky says. "And we may never have clinical evidence, because you can't easily do those kinds of experiments over a decade with people. But the more studies that come along showing that drinkers are less likely to have heart disease, the more consistency we have. And the more likely it becomes that there really is some sort of effect."

Let's look at some findings.

One of the main causes of heart disease and heart attacks is atherosclerosis—arteries clogged by hard, fatty deposits. Some studies seem to show that the more you drink, the less atherosclerosis you have, even if you drink to excess.

In Dr. Klatsky's study of alcohol and hospitalization, nondrinkers were hospitalized more often than even heavy drinkers for atherosclerosis-related symptoms like chest pain and heart attacks.

"The idea that heavier drinkers have less coronary blockage has been around since the turn of the century," Dr. Klatsky says. "Pathologists have said from way back how clean the blood vessels looked in heavy drinkers." And they're still saying that.

Researchers at Tufts-New England Medical Center, Boston, recently matched postmortem cross sections of heart arteries from people who had alcohol-related liver cirrhosis with artery sections from people of the same age and sex who did not have cirrhosis. Those with the liver disease showed much less narrowing of arteries and scar tissue formation, even when they had other risk factors like smoking, hypertension and a family history of heart disease (*Internal Medicine News,* June 15-30, 1982).

Researchers now know that drinking alcohol raises blood levels of high-density lipoproteins (HDL), blood fats thought to help prevent atherosclerosis and heart disease. But recently scientists have broken HDL into subgroups and found that apparently not all its forms are protective. HDL_2, the form raised by exercise, appears to be. But HDL_3, the form raised by alcohol, seems not to have a protective effect. William Haskell, Ph.D., associate professor of medicine at Stanford University, made that finding.

"You can't totally discount what appears to be a lower risk of heart disease with alcohol consumption, or that it may be due to an alteration in fat metabolism," Dr. Haskell says. "There may be a lot of other things going on that we haven't looked at yet that may result in some kind of beneficial influence."

Research seems to indicate that alcohol can also help stop red blood cells from clumping together and forming clots that can clog arteries.

Several years ago, research at the Medical College of Wisconsin in Milwaukee showed that even when they had as much artery blockage as nondrinkers, people who drank were less likely to go on to have a fatal heart attack. Since this seemed to be independent of the amount of narrowing of the arteries and hence, of blood fats, the researchers theorized that perhaps alcohol interfered with blood clotting. A recent English study supports that theory.

Researchers at Kings' College, London, checked the rate of blood clumping in volunteers, in each case before and after they drank a total of 25 ounces of white wine, ate a meal high in saturated fats, and had the wine along with their meal. They found wine alone had no inhibiting effect on blood clumping. The fatty meal alone increased blood clumping. But when the wine was taken along with the meal, much less clumping occurred (*Thrombosis Haemostas,* vol. 51, no. 1, 1984).

Alcohol may have another, very complex role in the cardiovascular system. It seems to affect the fluidity of cell membranes, changing the way cells absorb or release substances. One substance alcohol seems to affect is calcium, a mineral that plays an important role in blood vessel constriction, dilation and spasm. Alcohol affects both blood pressure and the incidence of stroke, says Dr. Altura, a leading researcher in this area.

"Some very preliminary research suggests that low amounts of alcohol might have an antispasmodic, or relaxing, effect on some blood vessels, particularly peripheral vessels," Dr. Altura says. But he adds many cautions. In some studies, even low amounts of alcohol constricted heart, brain and kidney blood vessels.

Most studies show that heavy drinkers tend to have higher blood pressure than normal. In one of Dr. Klatsky's studies, men having two or fewer drinks a day had about the same blood pressures as nondrinkers. Women drinking that same amount had slightly lower blood pressures. But men and women who took three to five drinks a day had blood pressures a few points higher than nondrinkers. And those taking six or more drinks a day had pressures up to ten points higher and twice as many readings over 160/95.

One very recent finding in alcohol research, Dr. Altura says, is that binge drinking can lead to stroke. "When alcohol concentration builds up to a certain point, blood vessels in the brain can actually rupture," he says.

What do we know about moderate alcohol use and the brain? Not much, admits Charles Golden, Ph.D., professor of medical psychology at the University of Nebraska, Omaha. "We do know it normally takes about ten years of steady abuse for obvious brain damage." The brain actually shrinks as if in a kind of speeded-up aging process that hurts the ability to reason and react. Sometimes these effects go away when a person stops drinking. Sometimes they're permanent.

"Some people, though, whom we can't fully identify, develop damage much faster and at lower levels of alcohol than most people," Dr. Golden says. "It's not so much the amount of alcohol that matters, but the individual's reaction to it. Brain damage could occur even with moderate drinking." People who seem to overreact to alcohol—who have extreme personality changes, blackouts or confusion with small amounts— might want to consider themselves susceptible, Dr. Golden says.

Researchers at the University of California at Los Angeles found that light social drinkers—people who said they drank an average of four times a week, typically having two or three drinks—did less well on cognitive functioning tests than nondrinkers, even when they were sober. Alcoholics usually do very poorly on these tests.

So how much is too much?

"There's a big difference between dealing with a patient one-on-one and making health pronouncements," says Dr.

Klatsky. "An individual doctor knows his patients and uses his judgment to come up with sound advice regarding alcohol use. I say that people who are already drinking two or fewer drinks a day and know they can control their intake need not change their habits. But it's much more difficult to say that people who don't drink should. Plenty of times they have good reasons they should not drink."

"I think the overriding message that has come out of these statistics is that there is a daily intake below which risk to health is minimal," Dr. Turner says.

"We've developed a very simple table—if you divide your body weight in pounds by 30, it gives you the number of ounces of 80-proof liquor you should not exceed daily. If you divide by 3, it gives you the number of ounces of beer. And if you divide by 9, it gives you the number of ounces of wine."

For a 150-pound man, that comes to 5 ounces of 80-proof liquor (about three shots), 50 ounces of beer (four 12-ounce cans), or 16 ounces of wine (about three 5-ounce glasses).

But other doctors are quite cautious. "There are just too many factors in those studies that have not been elucidated," Dr. Altura says. "I think it is dangerous to tell people that low doses of alcohol are beneficial. I think in the long term those low doses can accumulate and could create disastrous effects on the brain and the heart."

Another problem is that each person has his or her own sensitivity to alcohol and some people are quite sensitive, especially to early liver damage.

In Short . . .

● People who have two or fewer drinks a day seem to have less heart disease and illness in general than people who don't drink at all.

● Moderate drinkers may not necessarily be healthier *because* they drink. Other still-unknown factors could account for differences between these two groups.

● Even in small amounts, alcohol can cause liver and brain damage in sensitive people. It is difficult to know if you are vulnerable before symptoms arise. And in large amounts it can lead to alcoholism, a devastating disease.

- Keep in mind that many of alcohol's reported "benefits" can probably be attained in safer ways—by not smoking and by exercising, keeping your weight down, eating a low-fat diet and practicing other commonsense lifestyle habits.

Foods That Can Give You a Headache

She was a wealthy woman whose hobby was window-shopping. But suddenly her hobby became a headache, a daily throbbing migraine that threatened to cut short her fantasy buying sprees. Her doctor suspected it was all her sidewalk-pounding, putting a strain on her spine, which was telegraphing pain to her head. But before he prescribed a more sedentary pastime, he checked her eating habits. There he found a more likely culprit: the bag of candy she ate as she cruised the chic shops of Beverly Hills. It was chocolate that triggered her headaches.

He was a traveling salesman who scoffed at the idea that his migraines could be caused by something he ate. "It can't be food," he insisted. "I eat Mexican one night, at Bob's Big Boy another. I never eat the same thing." But when he grudgingly completed a food diary, he discovered that whether he was eating a burrito or a burger, he always had a salad heaped with fresh tomatoes. When he eliminated the tomatoes, the headaches went, too.

An estimated 40 million Americans suffer from chronic headaches, some that defy aspirin and cold compresses, some so debilitating their victims lose jobs and families. Many desperate headache sufferers turn to high-powered painkillers or biofeedback techniques. But these days, an increasing number are learning to spell relief D-I-E-T.

It's a controversial remedy. There is little scientific evidence linking headaches to food. That puts doctors like Seymour Diamond, M.D., in a curious bind. Dr. Diamond, founder of the renowned Diamond Headache Clinic in Chicago and the

National Migraine Foundation, has never been able to prove in the laboratory what he knows from his practice.

"As a researcher I have some doubts about the relationship of diet to headaches. As a clinician I have no doubts," he says. "Basically I'm a clinician who does research, so I have a very strong feeling that migraine sufferers are helped by diet—at least 25 to 30 percent of them are."

Not only migraine sufferers can look to a dietary remedy. Some tension and muscular headaches may signal masked food sensitivities and are easily remedied by a slight change in diet. So-called weekend headaches are often cured by moving up weekend breakfast times to prevent the drop in blood sugar that triggers the headache in the first place. There is even a way to eat that first bite of butter almond to avoid the dreaded "ice cream headache" and a nutritional prescription for the headache of Chinese restaurant syndrome.

Needless to say, there is no diet that cures them all, no medical advice as simple as, "Take two grapes and call me in the morning." Each remedy is as individual as the headache, so "The Antiheadache Diet" isn't a diet at all but a set of guidelines, based on the advice of experts, that will help you determine a diet remedy that works for you.

The Migraine Headache

You've just returned from a cocktail party where you gorged on great chunks of fine aged Cheddar, creamy Brie slathered on fresh French bread, handfuls of salted nuts and chocolate-covered petit fours. And maybe, just maybe, you drank a tad too much burgundy.

If you are susceptible to migraine headaches—severe vascular headaches that can leave you nauseated—you've just concocted a surfire recipe to bring one on. Everything you ate and drank has been identified as a migraine trigger. The wine (red in particular), the aged cheese and the chocolate all contain substances called amines, which can cause blood vessels to swell, triggering a headache. The nuts, salt and fresh-baked bread are also known to bring on migraines in people with sensitive vascular systems.

Does this mean that migraine sufferers have to avoid parties and party foods? Not necessarily. But they may have to alter their eating habits. Most headache experts have their own lists of "foods to avoid," but they agree that the best rule of thumb is: If it gives you a headache, don't eat it.

It's not scientific, admits Joan Miller, Ph.D., a headache expert from Atlanta. "But my feeling is that the scientific evidence isn't as important as, 'Does it work?' "

Even if you consult a professional, it still is largely up to you to unravel your own personal headache mystery. But it might help to know a list of the most common suspects. Along with the ones we've mentioned, these include soy sauce, meats cured with nitrites, caffeinated beverages, foods containing the flavor enhancer monosodium glutamate, dairy products, broad beans such as limas and navy beans, citrus fruits, tomatoes, onions, pork, herring and other seafood, fresh wheat and yeast products, licorice and vinegar, except the white variety.

Most headache experts advise eliminating the amine-containing foods and experimenting with the others, eating one food at a time to determine if it figures in your headache. Of course, the method isn't foolproof. Some headaches don't appear until up to a day or two after the offending food is eaten. Some headaches aren't triggered by one but by a combination of foods, or by food in tandem with stress.

"Many times you can get away with eating a certain food until you're under some stress, then the food plus the stress equals a migraine," says Dr. Miller, "I've had clients who've triggered a headache with a handful of peanuts eaten during a stressful time. Yet two weeks before they ate nuts and didn't get a headache."

Salt, like stress, is a subtle headache trigger. So says John Brainard, M.D., a surgeon from St. Paul, Minnesota, whose own migraines spurred him to write *Control of Migraines* (W.W. Norton & Co., 1977), the story of his dietary self-remedy.

Dr. Brainard noticed that when he ate salty foods, he was particularly susceptible to migraine. "Salt affects the blood vessels in such a way that it can make you very susceptible to other substances," he says.

The Food-Sensitivity Headache

She was 34 and for the last ten years of her life she had had a daily tension headache. At least, that's what her doctor called it. The other evidence was all there: temper outbursts, irritability, nervous tension, moodiness. The headache would go on for hours if she didn't take aspirin. Desperate, she sought help at the Institute of Health Psychology at North Texas State University, Denton.

There, psychologist Dan O'Banion, Ph.D., didn't discount the original diagnosis, but wasn't so sure her tension was psychological in origin. He placed her on an elimination diet, one that permitted her to eat only one food at a time. For the first time in a decade, the patient had several successive headache-free days—days, not coincidentally, when she didn't consume corn, wheat, milk products, cola drinks and tea.

"Hers was a tension headache," says Dr. O'Banion, "but the tension was caused by her food sensitivity. Much of the increased stress load on people like this is due to diet. Their bodies become toxic and it makes them susceptible to even small psychological problems."

Though relatively simple to pinpoint, food-sensitivity headaches aren't always simple to cure. Often the victims are sensitive to their favorite food. The fact is, the psychologist says, many food-sensitive people become addicted to the food they're sensitive to. They get a "high" when they eat it and crash when they don't. The headache they experience when they don't get their "food fix" is a symptom of withdrawal, Dr. O'Banion says. Some people even wake up several times a night, unable to sleep until they eat their particular addictive food.

The only diet remedy for this particular headache is similar to that for a migraine: Eat only fresh foods and use an elimination test to determine which foods trigger your particular headache. The food-withdrawal headache usually occurs two to three hours after the offending food is eaten, says Dr. O'Banion. You might have to suffer with it for several days, he warns, until you shake the addictive cycle.

The Hypoglycemic Headache

When the sugar content of the blood drops, blood vessels swell, causing vascular headaches such as migraines, says Dr. Diamond in a book he co-authored with Judi Diamond-Falk, *Advice from the Diamond Headache Clinic* (International Universities Press, 1982). These headaches can be avoided if you eat several small meals a day, have a protein snack before bed so your blood sugar doesn't dwindle by morning and avoid simple-carbohydrate, high-sugar foods that cause a rapid rise and fall in blood sugar levels.

The Hunger Headache

Similar to the hypoglycemic headache, this one is also caused by a drop in blood sugar, says Dr. Diamond. The remedy is simple: Eat at least three well-balanced meals a day.

The Hangover Headache

This one is avoidable. Simply don't drink to excess. But if you expect to overindulge, says Dr. Diamond, there is a way to lessen the pain. Eating fruit or honey, even drinking tomato juice, can reduce the impact of a hangover headache. Fructose helps the body metabolize ethyl alchol, he says.

The Caffeine and Caffeine-Withdrawal Headaches

This is a case of damned if you do and damned if you don't. Caffeine can cause a headache if you drink it and if you suddenly stop drinking it.

A strong stimulant, caffeine can make you so edgy you develop a tension headache. It can keep you awake, inviting the dull throb of fatigue. It can also raise your blood pressure, which can give you a dull, pounding headache or increase the frequency of your migraines.

Caffeine is also a vasoconstrictor—it makes your blood vessels contract. They can adapt quite readily to this semi-constricted state if you're a habitual caffeine drinker. But if you decide to go cold turkey, vessels swell, leaving you with a dull withdrawal headache that can be cured only by more caffeine—or time and a painkiller. The best remedy, says Dr. Diamond, is to gradually wean yourself from caffeine.

The Weekend Headache

You wake up blissfully late on Saturday morning only to find your day off marred by a headache. You suspect there's a voodoo doll somewhere with a pin in its head—and your name on it. No one is really sure what causes these weekend woes, but there are some likely culprits. If you don't eat breakfast at your regular weekday time, you could have a hunger headache. The remedy? Get up and eat something, even if you go right back to bed, says Dr. Diamond. Or you could be going through caffeine withdrawal, particularly if you restrict your coffee drinking to the office. You already know the remedy for that.

The Poor Nutrition Headache

Many headache sufferers simply don't take good care of themselves, says Dr. Miller. Many bear an uncanny resemblance to the typical Type A personality: busy fussbudgets who'll forgo meals and family affairs to work, work, work. The missed meals often mean a loss of the B-complex vitamins, which can leave them edgy and prone to headaches. "Headache sufferers tend not to connect their headaches to anything they do," she says. "Most need nutritional counseling. They're used to curing everything with a pill. They need to know that the food they eat has something to do with their bodies."

The best cure for this headache is prevention, Dr. Miller says. A well-balanced diet and evenly spaced meals—that means no snack on the run—will keep your body healthy and the headaches away.

The Hot Dog Headache

The culprit isn't that familiar *cuisine de ballpark* per se, it's the nitrites used in the curing process, which give the meat that appetizing red color. Nitrites are found in everything from lunch meat to bacon and there is a cure for this cure. Just add cured meats to your "foods to avoid" list.

Chinese Restaurant Syndrome

Some people don't get hungry an hour after eating Chinese food, they get a headache. It's not the *moo goo gai pan* but the monosodium glutamate (MSG) that triggers this reaction, which also includes a feeling of tightness in the chest and a burning sensation in the face, neck and torso. You don't have to give up chinese food. Many restaurants don't add this flavor enhancer and most would be happy to leave it out of your dish if you ask.

According to Rosemary Dudley, executive vice president of the Migraine Foundation of Canada, MSG headaches are most pronounced if you eat on an empty stomach, so before your Chinese dinner, eat a roll or a salad. Also, try to avoid starting your meal with soup, which can contain more of this nasty substance than the vegetable and meat dishes you eat later on.

Be forewarned: MSG is also used in some processed and prepared foods. If you don't already read food labels, start. You might save yourself a headache later on.

The Ice Cream Headache

You've just taken a big bite of butter almond and an intense, dull pain radiates throughout your head. Not what you had in mind, was it? Exactly what causes an ice cream headache isn't known. But, according to Dr. Diamond, the pain may be a response of the warm tissues of the mouth to the cold substance. Two nerves there carry impulses—including pain—to the head, which explains why the headache is generalized in the head and throat.

If you're a victim, there's a way to eat ice cream that won't bring on a headache. Simply allow small amounts of ice cream, or other cold substances, to melt or warm up in the mouth so that the mouth cools slowly, advises Dr. Diamond.

Foods for the Headache-Prone

This is the proverbial good news, foods that seem relatively safe for most headache sufferers. The selection was culled from food lists provided by Dr. Diamond, Gunnar

Heuser, M.D., Ph.D., of the Beverly Hills Headache and Pain Medical Group, and Dr. Brainard.

Dairy Products • Cottage cheese, cream cheese, yogurt (½ cup). Other cheeses may be tolerated if they are cooked in a dish such as lasagna.

Desserts • Cakes, cookies, fruit pies, gelatin, tapioca. (Avoid fresh yeast-raised products or those containing chocolate, nuts or raisins.)

Fruit • Apples, apricots, bananas (½ a day), blueberries, cherries, citrus fruits (½ cup a day), cranberries, grapes, peaches, pears.

Meat • Beef, chicken, duck, lamb, turkey, veal.

Vegetables • Artichokes, asparagus, beets, broccoli, carrots, cauliflower, celery, cucumbers, eggplant, green beans, leafy greens, mushrooms, parsnips, peas, potatoes, sprouts.

Miscellaneous • Commercial bread, carob, eggs, homemade salad dressings (or commercial dressings in small amounts), homemade soups, salt-free snacks.

The Fiber Breakthrough

Years ago nutritional scientists viewed dietary fiber the way they once viewed "vitamin B": It was supposed to be a single substance with a single function that barely got a niche in the medical mind.

But vitamin B has become B complex, and dietary fiber (the roughage of yesteryear) is now surprising a lot of people with a complexity of its own.

The American Cancer Society and the National Cancer Institute now want more fiber in our diets. The food industry embraces it. The popular press hails it. And research labs around the world add support to decade-old hypotheses that it may help prevent obesity, colon cancer, heart disease, gallstones, irritable bowel syndrome, diverticulosis and diabetic conditions.

With all this fuss, it's become clear that dietary fiber is more diverse in its forms and biological effects than anyone ever imagined. And among medical people, fiber's potential for promoting health has never seemed greater. The F complex has arrived.

"Nowadays most nutritionists realize that dietary fiber is multifaceted," says Peter J. Van Soest, Ph.D., a leading fiber researcher at Cornell University. "They know that it's not just one thing, but a collection of things—a variety of elements with a variety of functions."

This latter-day insight into fiber's true nature has already helped give the lie to some old ideas on the subject. False: "Bran" is synonymous with "fiber." False: All fiber is fibrous, or stringy. False: All fiber tastes the same.

The fallacies are more apparent as soon as you realize that dietary fiber is actually the indigestible remnants of plant cells (mostly cell walls)—remnants that come in at least six types and show up in everything from bulgur to blueberries. And the difference in physiological impact among these six classes of fiber can be as vast as that between penicillin and spring water.

Cellulose • This is the most prevalent fiber and probably comes closest to the hoary notions of what fiber ought to be. It is indeed fibrous, softens the stool and abounds in all the expected places—fruits, vegetables, bran, whole meal bread and beans.

But you'll find it in some unlikely places, too—nuts and seeds—and it does more than the old notions suggest. It increases the bulk of intestinal waste and eases it quickly through the colon. All of which means, of course, that it prevents constipation, but some investigators say that these actions may dilute and flush cancer-causing toxins out of the intestinal tract. Research also indicates that cellulose may help level out glucose in the blood and—because of its ability to fill you up without fattening you out—curb weight gain.

One thing it can't do, however, is lower your cholesterol. That's a function reserved for other kinds of fiber.

Hemicellulose • The name is a misnomer—it's not half cellulose. It has a chemical character all its own, but usually shows up wherever cellulose is and shares some of its traits. Hemicellulose, too, may help relieve constipation, water down carcinogens in the bowel and aid in weight reduction. And, like cellulose, it has no known effect on cholesterol.

Pectin • This kind of fiber may be better than any other kind at pushing down cholesterol levels.

"For some reason, water-holding fiber like cellulose has no influence on serum cholesterol levels," says David Kritchevsky, Ph.D., biochemist and coeditor of *Dietary Fiber in Health and Disease* (Plenum Press, 1982). "But water-soluble fibers like pectin and gums can reduce cholesterol."

But then pectin doesn't have a celluloselike influence on the stool. It can do nothing to deter constipation.

Just the same, researchers have been looking into the possibility that pectin can aid the elimination of bile acids through the intestinal tract, short-circuiting the development of gallstones and colon cancer. Common sources of pectin: apples, citrus fruits, grapes, berries and—contrary to fiber lore—bran.

Gums and Mucilages • You eat these sticky fibers every day without even realizing it, for you usually encounter them as plant-derived thickening agents in everything from ketchup to store-bought cookies.

But invesigators have dicovered that gums, at least, can do far more than give condiments body. They've found that locust-bean gum, karaya gum, guar gum, oat gum and others can lower cholesterol significantly. And they've shown that a few gums can even help diabetics handle blood sugar better.

"There's a lot of scientific excitement surrounding the gum fibers," one researcher told us. "They seem to be more effective in the treatment of diabetics than some other fibers, and they're certainly more palatable than the water-soluble ones."

Lignin ● The main talent of this type of fiber is escorting bile acids and cholesterol out of the intestines. There's even some evidence that it may prevent the formation of gallstones. You'll find high proportions of it in cereals, bran, whole meal flour, raspberries, strawberries, brussels sprouts, cabbage, spinach, kale, parsley and tomatoes. The more mature the vegetable, the greater the lignin content.

But lignin, pectin, gum or some other type of fiber isn't exactly the kind of thing you'll find in quart jars on your grocer's shelf. Nature has already packaged them in countless foods, in combinations that can produce a startling array of physiological changes. And it's these fiber foods, not the fiber types, that researchers have scrutinized the most. Here's a rundown of fact and fable concerning some of these top fiber sources:

Bran ● This flaky remnant of grains is one of the world's richest sources of dietary fiber. (Not *the* richest because the raspberry, for one, has it beat.) And it contains not one, but several types of fiber, including cellulose, hemicellulose and pectin. But the generalizations about bran can stop right there, for there are too many discrete brans, each with its own personality.

Wheat bran has a reputation for relieving constipation, and research concurs (though a recent study indicates that corn bran may be even better at solving this problem). And evidence suggests that wheat bran may help modulate glucose levels in diabetics and reduce the symptoms of diverticulosis, an intestinal disorder.

A controversy is brewing, however, over whether your morning bowl of wheat bran can have a positive effect on cholesterol. Most of the evidence has said no, but the latest study on the subject begs to differ. Investigators in Sweden added concentrated wheat bran to the diets of patients with high cholesterol levels, then monitored the effects. Surprise: The patient's LDL (low-density lipoprotein) and VLDL (very low-density lipoprotein) cholesterol (the harmful kinds) decreased slightly, and HDL (high-density lipoprotein) cholesterol (the beneficial kind) increased dramatically.

There's no such controversy, though, surrounding the cholesterol-lowering effects of oat bran. James W. Anderson,

M.D., of the University of Kentucky in Lexington, has seen to that. He put oat bran on the nutritional map when he demonstrated in several studies that adding oat bran to the diet can reduce cholesterol levels drastically. In one such experiment involving men with elevated cholesterol, the reduction averaged 13 percent.

On top of that, says Dr. Anderson, oat bran is tastier than a lot of other fiber-rich fare. "Oat bran is palatable as a hot cereal and can be incorporated into muffins, breads and other prepared foods," he says.

But it would be a mistake to expect oat bran to relieve constipation. It's rich in water-soluble fiber, which generally has no effect on bowel movements.

Corn bran, however, is more versatile. It not only can ease the symptoms of constipation, but also can lower LDL cholesterol, reduce the blood fats known as triglycerides and perhaps improve the body's ability to handle glucose, or blood sugar. This latter capability was suggested by a study indicating that a daily intake of as little as 26 grams (less than an ounce) of corn bran could improve people's scores on glucose-tolerance tests.

Legumes ● Peas, soybeans, lentils, chick-peas—these and their kin have high fiber content, but few people realize just how high. They actually outdo most fruits and vegetables. Canned baked beans, for example, register over 7 grams of dietary fiber per 100 grams of beans (about 3½ ounces), while cooked broccoli weighs in at around 4 and cooked cabbage at just under 3.

Much of this fiber is water-soluble, which, as you might guess, makes legumes likely agents for lowering cholesterol. And research is slowly confirming this crucial capability. Dr. Anderson and a colleague, for example, recently discovered that they could lower serum cholesterol in men with excessive cholesterol levels by adding about four ounces of pinto and navy beans to the men's daily meals. Total cholesterol dropped a remarkable 19 percent.

"While bean-supplemented diets were as effective as oat bran-supplemented diets in lowering serum cholesterol concentrations," the investigators say, "oat bran was better tolerated [fewer problems like intestinal gas] by our patients" (*Unconventional Sources of Dietary Fiber,* American Chemical Society, 1983). But can legumes help ease the problem of constipation? Probably not. Can they help control glucose levels? Probably, especially if the legumes happen to be soybeans. Researchers have been reporting that both soy hulls and a powdered soy supplement can improve glucose tolerance.

Vegetables and Fruit • Scientists have tested very few of these for fiberlike feats of physiology, though it's obvious that these foods contain types of fiber known to do a lot of healthful deeds. Researchers instead have busied themselves with measuring the fiber constituents and total fiber content of these edibles—and overturned some misconceptions in the process.

For example, we now know that "vegetable fiber" isn't all cellulose. Often, as in the case of green beans and brussels sprouts, it's not even *mostly* cellulose. Similarly, "fruit fiber" isn't 100 percent pectin, though it usually has a high percentage of that fiber. Cellulose, lignin and other types are in the mix, too.

And, as you may already know, the total fiber content of a fruit or vegetable can surprise you. The vegetables with the biggest fiber ratings, for example, include sweet corn, parsnips, carrots, potatoes and peas. And among the highest ranking fruits are raspberries, pears, strawberries and guavas. Ounce for ounce, a peach has more fiber in it than a turnip does, cherries more than a green pepper, and carrots more than cabbage.

So how much fiber should you be eating?

Some Africans, known for lower incidence of degenerative diseases, consume as much as 150 grams (about 5^1/$_3$ ounces) of fiber a day. Intake in Europe and North America, where such diseases are rampant, is 25 grams or less a day, with many people getting as little as 10 grams.

Experts don't suggest that Americans should match the high fiber intake of Africans, but they do agree that most people aren't getting enough fiber. Unfortunately, there's no RDA for fiber and very little data on optimum amounts. More and more researchers, though, are venturing some concrete recommendations based on the evidence that does exist. John H. Cummings, M.D., a noted fiber expert in England, recently advocated a fiber intake for adults of 30 grams (about one ounce) a day. And other investigators have echoed this suggestion.

"We really don't know what the optimum intake of dietary fiber should be," says Dr. Van Soest. "It is possible to get some positive benefits from fiber at the 30- to 40-gram mark, but you have to adjust the amount to what is comfortable for your own body."

But even this amount is far more than many Americans are getting, so some authorities have been coupling their fiber recommendations with some sound advice. Increase your fiber intake slowly, they say, to give your system time to adjust, gradually incorporating a variety of fibers from a variety of naturally occurring sources.

After all, you have a vast F complex to choose from.

FINDING THE FIBER YOU NEED

Fiber Type	Probable Functions	Food Sources	
Cellulose	Relieves constipation, counteracts carcinogens in the intestinal tract, modulates glucose, curbs weight gain.	Apples Bran and whole grain cereals Brazil nuts Brussels sprouts Carrots Lima beans	Peanuts Pears Peas Rhubarb Whole wheat flour
Hemicellulose	Relieves constipation, counteracts carcinogens in the intestinal tract, curbs weight gain.	Apples Bananas Beets Bran and whole grain cereals	Green beans Radishes Sweet corn

FINDING THE FIBER YOU NEED
—Continued

Fiber Type	Probable Functions	Food Sources	
Pectin	Lowers cholesterol, counters bile acids in the intestinal tract. Offers protection against colon cancer and gallstone formation.	Apples Bananas Beets Carrots	Okra Oranges Potatoes
Gums/ Mucilages	Lower cholesterol, modulate glucose levels.	Dried beans Oat bran Oatmeal	
Lignin	Escorts bile acids and cholesterol out of the intestines. Offers protection against colon cancer and gallstone formation.	Bran and whole grain cereals Brazil nuts Cabbage Peaches Peanuts	Pears Peas Strawberries Tomatoes

SOURCES: Adapted from
"Topics in Dietary Fiber," A Report of the Cornell University Agricultural Experiment Station, ed. G.A. Spiller (New York: Plenum Press, 1978).
"Fiber Analysis Tables," A Report of Research of the Cornell University Agricultural Experiment Station, *American Journal of Clinical Nutrition*, October, 1979.

Best Fitness
Ideas for 1985

Super Nutrition
for Super Performance

When Martina Navratilova won the U.S. Open tennis tournament in 1983, she didn't thank just her coaches. Included in the kudos was Robert Haas, Ph.D., the sports nutritionist who redesigned her diet and whom she credits with helping her to "peak performance."

Many world-class athletes are discovering that what they put in their mouths may affect their performances as much as the work they put into their training programs.

Should *recreational* athletes be equally concerned about nutrition? Your performance in the town race or company fun run may not have stakes as high as the U.S. Open, but if competing well is important to you, then yes, nutrition does count. Even if you exercise but don't compete, good nutrition can spur you on to higher energy levels and help you stay cool through the hot summer.

By good nutrition, sports nutritionists usually mean avoiding excessive fats and calories and getting enough of the right vitamins and minerals, either through the foods you eat or by supplementation.

In recent years supplementation to improve performance has gotten a bad name, probably because of such useless and possibly dangerous items as the *non*vitamin B_{15}. But legitimate vitamin and mineral supplements have been proven to enhance stamina and energy—key measures of performance.

One of the best experiments that studied the effect of vitamin and mineral supplementation on athletic performance was conducted by Michael Colgan, Ph.D., of the Colgan Nutritional Institute, Carlsbad, California. Dr. Colgan believes that even so-called balanced diets are probably lacking when it comes to basic nutrients—and he tested athletes to back up his theories.

Dr. Colgan divided ten experienced marathon runners between the ages of 28 and 44 into two groups. Half the runners were given complete vitamin and mineral supplements; the other half got lookalike placebo pills. Neither Dr. Colgan nor the runners knew which marathoners were really taking the vitamins. This double-blind method of research assures scientists of an unbiased outcome.

After six months, the runners taking supplements made *big* improvements in their running times—an average improvement of 17 minutes and 44 seconds. The runners who weren't supplemented had some improvement—after all, they were in training—but it was much less, averaging only 6 minutes and 43 seconds.

Dr. Colgan's athletes used a multivitamin and mineral supplement that contained vitamins A, B complex, C, D and E and the minerals zinc, iron, calcium, magnesium, manganese, phosphorus, potassium, copper, molybdenum, chromium, selenium and iodine. It's his belief that a wide range of supplements, taken over at least three to six months, is what's needed to affect athletic performance.

Other studies concerning athletic performance have looked at individual vitamins and minerals. One of the most important groups of vitamins for exercisers is the B complex. While these vitamins work as a group to enhance energy and strength, a few B vitamins have been studied separately.

Daphne Roe, M.D., a professor of nutrition at Cornell University in Ithaca, New York, found that active people need significantly higher amounts of riboflavin (vitamin B_2) than people who don't exercise regularly. She thinks that exercisers may need twice the Recommended Dietary Allowance (RDA) of 1.2 milligrams daily.

Dr. Haas says riboflavin is especially important for women athletes. In his book *Eat to Win* (Rawson Associates, 1983), Dr. Haas says riboflavin helps women build and maintain strong muscle fiber.

Iron, of course, is also an energy booster for athletes. A Swedish study comparing two groups of athletes working out on exercise bikes found that the group supplemented with iron had four times more improvement in work performance than the nonsupplemented group.

Although you may be more concerned with the effect vitamins and minerals have on your exercise *performance*, certain nutrients can also help keep you cool during hot summer months.

If you want to beat the heat, tops on your list should be potassium and magnesium. These minerals are called electrolytes, and they're vital to your cooling system. Your body loses electrolytes when you perspire during exercise, so it's important to replace them.

One nutrient you *don't* need to replace, however, is salt. "Salt intake isn't very important and, in fact, may be negative," says George Jessup, Ph.D., a physical fitness expert at Texas A&M University's Human Performance Laboratory.

Dr. Jessup says the naturally occurring salt in many water supplies is high enough that very few people need extra salt to meet their bodies' requirements. You'll especially want to avoid salt tablets, which can actually accelerate sweating and cause dehydration.

On the plus side, extra vitamin C may help keep you cooler while you exercise. That's been proven by experiments among mine workers in South Africa. When compared with a group not taking vitamin C, a supplemented group had consistently lower body temperatures. Other experiments in the southern U.S. also showed vitamin C's ability to temper heat stress.

How to Get
Back in Shape

This story is for those of you who can't remember the last time you did anything more physically demanding than hike up your trousers or wrestle with your conscience—but who also feel anxious to do something about it.

For that purpose we've put together a primer on adult exercise, an informal A-B-C in seven steps that can help get you out of the starting blocks and back in the running. Included are tips on finding the right "soft" exercise, on staying motivated and on reacquainting yourself with long-neglected muscles. Our advice won't prepare you for a ten-kilometer race, but it might help you lead a more active, more enjoyable life.

Why should you think about a fitness program at this stage in your life? For two reasons. First, physiologists believe that exercise is the best natural age-reversing agent ever known. And second, they know that it's never too late to benefit from working out. Based on talks with a variety of exercise experts, here are some tips for getting started:

STEP 1: Get a complete physical examination ● You may be eager to start your new exercise program right away, but it would be foolish to rush out, buy a pair of striped sneakers and begin walking or jogging at dawn. All of the fitness specialists we spoke with emphasized the importance of a physical for people who've been "out of action" for years. Even though one of the goals of fitness is to rely on doctors as little as possible, an adult's exercise program should start in the doctor's office. Says Philadelphia clinical nutritionist Steven H. Small, D.M.D., "We recommend that anyone who is over 40 or out of shape undergo a complete physical before starting any fitness program."

There are two specific tests you should ask your doctor for. The first is an electrocardiogram, which measures the regularity of your heartbeat and displays the information on a graph for the doctor to see. The second is a step test (or some other comparable aerobic stress test), during which you spend five minutes putting your feet up on a step stool one at a time. The doctor will take your pulse before and after the test; the lower your heart rate afterward the more exercise your body can handle.

Beyond that, a physical can help you tailor a fitness program to your needs. The doctor will probably want to know what activities you used to enjoy or would like to take up, and what your health goals are. If your doctor says you shouldn't exercise, one fitness coach says, ask him why.

STEP 2: Be patient, go slow and don't "redline" yourself ● In other words, know your limits and don't exceed them. If you own a car with a tachometer, you know all about rpms, or the number of revolutions the engine makes per minute. You also know about the red danger zone at the high end of the dial, indicating that the engine is turning too fast and might come apart. It's the same way with your heart. It shouldn't exceed a certain beat-per-minute level.

The accepted formula for figuring your own maximum heart rate is to subtract your age from 220. If you are 55 years old, then, your redline zone begins at about 165. But that doesn't mean that you should push your heart that far. Dr. Small says that adult beginners should stay within 60 to 65 percent of their maximum heart rate. On the other hand, James A. Blumenthal, Ph.D., of the Duke University Preventive Approach to Cardiology program (DUPAC) says that his older patients often reach 70 to 85 percent of their maximum rate safely.

"Safely" is the key word. "The first thing I tell people is to know your age," says Ben E. Benjamin, Ph.D., a sports-medicine expert and the author of *Listen to Your Pain* (Penguin Books, 1983). "Don't try right away to do things that you used to do. Start very slowly and go especially slowly when you try things that you haven't done for years. A lot of people try to come back too fast."

STEP 3: Become aware of your own body ● Many adults lose touch with their own bodies. They may look at their reflections every day, but they don't necessarily see the gradual decline of their posture or the slow shrinking of their range of motion. Grace Hill, an exercise instructor in Hanover, New Hampshire, has noticed that when she tells her older students to reach up as far as they can, many of them lift their arms only as high as their ears. It's not that they can't go higher. They just aren't aware of where their arms are.

"The first thing I do is to draw people's attention to their own bodies," Mrs. Hill told us. "A lot of people have become oblivious to their bodies. They've lost their kinesthetic sense—the sense of how their bodies move and feel. They have to be reeducated. We use mirrors so that people can see what they're doing."

Yoga and fitness therapist Gopal Bello, a staff member at a health clinic in St. Johnsbury, Vermont, feels the same way. He tells his students to stand in front of a mirror and candidly assess their posture. Does the head slump forward? Is one shoulder higher than the other? Are the feet parallel? There's no such thing as good fitness without good posture, Bello says.

People also tend to lose awareness of their own breathing. "In the effort of trying to begin exercising," Mrs. Hill says, "most people unconsciously hold their breath. A good teacher reminds her students about breathing. You can't have endurance without it."

STEP 4: Choose "soft" exercises • When the experts recommend exercises for people past age 45 or 50, they rule out contact sports of any kind. They look for soft exercises that build up the body without punishing it.

"Water walking" is one of the most intriguing soft exercises we've heard of. It doesn't refer to any biblical miracle. It refers to walking, rather than swimming, in a pool. At DUPAC, older people exercise by walking laps in a four-foot-deep pool. Walking through water is a lot more strenuous than walking through air, but the buoyancy of the water all but eliminates the impact of the heel on the bottom of the pool. Not that there's anything wrong with swimming. Swimming gently puts every muscle in the body to work, and it's recommended by virtually all fitness experts. Bicycle riding, either stationary or mobile, is another respected soft exercise.

Rebounding is another recently developed soft exercise. Bouncing on one of those mini-trampolines that are about four feet wide and stand about six or seven inches above the floor is something of a fad, but people say it's a novel, low-impact way to jog in place.

Along with the right exercises, a person should know which exercises to avoid. University of Wisconsin dance professor Judy Alter claims that many traditional exercises are not only ineffective but also harmful. She points out "six don'ts" of calisthenics: bouncing, joint locking, arching, swinging, fast exercising and overbending the joints. All of them, she says, can harm muscles or joints.

Whenever you bend over to touch your toes and then bob up and down—that's bouncing. It can cause some muscle fibers to tear. Joint locking occurs when you hold your arm or leg rigid by extending the joint too far. Arching just means arching your back or neck backwards, as in a gymnastic back bend.

Swinging refers to exercises like jumping jacks where the motion of the exercise depends on momentum and your muscles are mostly passive. The potential harm comes when you suddenly reverse the direction of your arms or legs. Fast exercise refers to rushing through a strengthening exercise and not giving yourself the chance to feel the exercise strengthen your muscles. Overbending the joints is what happens when you do a deep bend so deep that your buttocks touch your heels. It puts tremendous stress on the ligaments in the knee.

One rule of thumb: If you feel pain, stop, especially when you're confronted by what Ms. Alter calls "ouch" pain. "When teachers or coaches say, 'If it hurts, it's good for you,' they are wrong," she says in her book *Surviving Exercise* (Houghton Mifflin, 1983). A sharp, stinging pain—the kind that makes you say "ouch!"—means that what you're doing is either unsafe or too strenuous or both.

STEP 5: Learn to "seduce" yourself ● One of the major obstacles to a new fitness program is inertia. It's the universal force that keeps you from getting out of bed in the morning and donning your sweat suit. Kelly Kessing, a staffer at Dr. Small's clinic in Philadelphia, recommends this strategy for outwitting inertia.

"You've got to seduce yourself into going out there," she says. "For instance, if the idea of walking intimidates you, just don't tell yourself that you're going for a walk. Don't pressure yourself. Put on your sweat shirt and your shoes. Tell yourself, 'Maybe I'll go for a walk, and maybe I won't.' Even if you still don't go for a walk, at least you'll have been up and moving for a few minutes."

If you're still intimidated, break the job down into smaller chunks and tackle one chunk at a time. "Walk 10 minutes six days in a row instead of 60 minutes one day a week," Ms. Kessing says. "And if at first you don't succeed, forgive yourself and start over."

STEP 6: Find the right program ● When shopping for a fitness center, look for a place that has treadmills and other monitoring devices. And look for a coach who won't mind answering your questions about aches and pains, clothes and shoes, liniments and hot pads. "A compassionate coach can give a person peace of mind," Ms. Kessing says.

STEP 7: Remind yourself that it's never too late to benefit from physical exercise ● Dr. Blumenthal's experiments at Duke University showed that older people can reverse a weak physique to some extent. His group of 24 people over age 65 exercised on stationary bicycles for 30 minutes, three times a week for 12 weeks. By program end they had lowered their heart rates and recovered a degree of aerobic capacity they hadn't felt in years.

"There's some controversy as to whether older people can improve their cardiovascular health," Dr. Blumenthal told us." "Our evidence is that they can to a certain degree."

Fitness therapist Bello agrees that older people should be more optimistic. "People very often feel that they just can't get better. They take it as given that they won't be able to do the things they used to do. But we've found that people can recover a lot of the range of motion they used to have."

The Stars and Your Health

Not the heavenly but the Hollywood kind.
The 1985 Annual looks at their diets, fitness
programs and shape-up plans, then grades
them and reports on what they can do for *you*.

Yes, Jane Fonda is beautiful and James Coco is a stitch. But are these people qualified to be instructing us on our health?

That's a good question. Jane Fonda's workout book has

already sold over 1,300,000 copies, and Coco's diet book is fast following in its footsteps. If these books are too far off the mark, a lot of us are in a lot of trouble.

Not all *scientists* are 100 percent happy about these entertainers treading on the fitness turf, but at least some have been able to view the invasion positively. For example, physiology professor Barbara Drinkwater, Ph.D., of the University of Washington, recently told *Physician and Sportsmedicine* that perhaps a "pat on the back" should be given to these celebrities for making "an effort to reach the public with reasonably accurate and useful information." And Leroy H. Getchell, Ph.D., of the Human Performance Laboratory at Ball State University, agreed: "I'm not against celebrity books. Some of them aren't bad, and besides, if you put *me* on the cover of a book, it'd never sell."

So without further ado, here's a look at the "guts" of what some of these celebrity-authored health books have to say.

The James Coco Diet
by James Coco
(Bantam Books, $13.95)

James Coco was so heavy while playing the part of Sancho Panza in *The Man of La Mancha* that he nearly crippled his donkey. That's the sort of bittersweet humor you get in *The James Coco Diet* (about 110 pages' worth, in fact). But once you get to the book's punchline, you find it's a no-nonsense, 700-calorie-a-day plan devised by Gerard J. Musante, Ph.D., director of a weight-loss center known as Structure House in Durham, North Carolina.

And with this diet, "structure" is the word. After 21 days of 700 calories a day, you step up to 1,000 per day for a week, followed by 1,200 per day for another week, followed by 1,800 a day for as many weeks as it takes you to reach your desired weight.

And what then? A "maintenance level" of calories calculated by multiplying your desired weight by 15 if you're a man, 12 if you're a woman.

"Obesity is a very personal problem, different for every single individual," Dr. Musante writes in his introduction, but there are certain common elements. Overweight people tend to eat out of sheer habit, out of boredom and due to stress. Habit (because of his Italian upbringing) and stress (because of his business) were Jimmy's two biggest problems, so that's what he and Dr. Musante worked on. Having seesawed his way up and down between 305 and 215 more times than he'd care to remember, he now weighs a permanent 205 and has never looked or felt better in his life.

The foods responsible? "Most diets are for the birds. My diet is for human beings," Jimmy brags in his preface. And it's not an idle boast. The menus offered in this book are varied, good-tasting and nutritious. There's nothing revolutionary about them, but in large measure that's their strength. They're rooted in basic and healthful foods. Our only bone to pick with *The James Coco Diet* is that pages devoted to show-biz anecdotes might have been better spent impressing on readers the weight-loss advantages of regular physical exercise. Seven hundred calories a day is not a lot. And though the diet calls for a daily vitamin supplement, a more healthful approach would be to take more calories in but put more calories out.

All in all, though, a good effort. We'll give Jim 3 (out of a possible 4) stars.

Richard Simmons' Better Body Book
by Richard Simmons
(Warner Books, $16.50)

If you can stand Richard's curls and cuteness, this book can give you a decent anatomy lesson. Richard's account of cellulite is one of the more imaginative we've encountered. "In people who have loose, weak muscles . . . there are no zoning laws. Fat looks lumpy and bumpy because it has spread out into suburbs, built a few high rises here and there and run all over your interior map without an architect."

Richard has an interesting viewpoint on whether or not to count while you do his exercises (better simply to do what you can, listening to your body and stopping when you begin to feel pain, he says). His approach to dieting is equally easygoing: Life's too short to deprive yourself totally, so splurge when you must, but make amends accordingly.

We have only one real gripe with Simmons' *Better*

Body Book, and it's a gripe that applies to many of the other "spot-exercise" books like it: There's not enough sustained heavy breathing. Richard at one point actually makes the erroneous statement that "aerobic exercise does not necessarily help you lose weight," when in fact, it's the *best* way of losing weight. Per amount of time spent, exercise that sustains a "target heart rate" (a figure you can determine by subtracting your age from 220 and then multiplying that number by 0.70) burns calories faster than any spot-reducing exercises.

Taken as a whole, though, *Richard Simmons' Better Body Book* is a step in the right direction toward a better body. Give Richard 3 stars.

Jane Fonda's Workout Book
by Jane Fonda
(Simon & Schuster, $19.95)

This is the book that most of the others have tried to match, and it's easy to see why. It's good. Jane is very up-front about the degree of commitment a top-notch fitness program requires ("There are no shortcuts," she warns), but she's also straightforward about the rewards of such a commitment. Fitness can help you find who and what you really are, Jane says. Once a body-abuser herself (diet pills, junk food, no exercise), she began finding that the more "good things" she did for herself (starting with ballet), the less she needed "the bad things." Her routine now, at age 46, is to work out for at least 40 minutes every day (usually in the morning) and to be prudent but not obsessed about what she eats. "Call off the fight and accept food as a life-giving friend," she says. And the way to do that? She lays down some basic rules:

1. Substitute low-fat foods for high-fat foods.
2. Cut down on meat.
3. Avoid salt and salty foods.
4. Cut down on sugar.
5. Emphasize whole grains, wheat germ, wheat bran and sprouts.
6. Beware of alcohol.

7. Snack on fresh fruits and vegetables, raw nuts, sesame seeds and yogurt.

Jane recommends making these rules a family affair, not just a personal fitness regimen, and she's a big believer in making breakfast the largest meal of the day. She's come up with a great substitute for coffee that she uses as an afternoon energizer (several tablespoons of brewer's yeast dissolved in a cup of hot water with a dash of cayenne or pepper for some zip), and she will often accompany it with a piece of fresh fruit.

As for the workout section of the book, it's divided into two sections (one for beginners, one for advanced). While both programs are good for improving muscle tone and flexibility, they do (like the Simmons program) fall a bit short in the area of aerobics. Jane has you concentrating on your cardiovascular conditioning for only several minutes out of a 40-minute routine. For purposes of both a healthier heart *and* greater weight loss, we'd advise lengthening this segment to at least 15 minutes.

All in all, though, it's a realistic, sincere and inspirational introduction to the joys of becoming physically fit. Give Jane 3½ stars.

The Body Principal
by Victoria Principal
(Simon & Schuster, $16.95)

Victoria's approach might be different from Jane Fonda's, but her message (and her physique) is pretty much the same: Make exercise as basic a part of your life as eating and sleeping and you've got fitness under control.

Jane likes to get her workout first thing in the morning; Victoria prefers to get hers all day long—in bits and pieces. She'll do modified push-ups in the ladies' room, using the sink. She'll do chestbuilders while getting her hair done for *Dallas*. By day's end she'll have gotten to all parts of her body.

And what a body. As with Jane Fonda, Victoria Principal is living proof of what a commitment to exercise can do. Her thoughts on nutrition also are good (she simply cuts out foods she knows are bad—oils, butter, sugar, salt and alcohol—and eats freely of foods she knows are good—vegetables, chicken, fish, low-fat dairy products, whole grain foods and fruit). And like Jane, she's a big believer in a hearty breakfast.

Any weaknesses to the book? Only that Victoria works harder on her body than most of her book lets on. No one looks *that* good doing just 20 minutes of light 'n' easy exercises a day. Not until her second-to-last chapter does Victoria admit to working out with weights or weight machines from one to three times a week, and by the looks of her muscles, we'd have to guess it's closer to three.

But *The Body Principal* is a good book, nonetheless. Sincere, scientifically accurate and sensible to the point of being worth 3½ stars. We wish we could say the same for Linda Evans' effort.

Linda Evans' Beauty and Exercise Book
by Linda Evans
(Simon & Schuster, $9.95)

Linda no doubt means well in revealing what we're told are her "personal secrets" for beauty and good health, but for the most part she'd have done as well to keep these secrets to herself. The other books we've looked at have been commendably rooted in reality, but this one is mired in misconceptions. Linda talks about avoiding carbohydrates to lose weight, massaging away fat and pulling on hair to thicken it. You find yourself wondering how Linda has managed, via these "secrets," to look as good as she does. She skirts the issue of requiring a certain amount of no-nonsense exercise to stay fit (preferring instead to talk about pushing fat away with rolling pins). And her section on diet offers advice no more concrete than to figure out why you overeat and vow not to. If the book could be said to have a purpose, it would be only to show us that, yes, the pie-in-the-sky health book is still possible (getting harder all the time, but still possible). Linda spends more time talking about how to apply makeup than she does on how to apply sound exercise or nutritional principals. Miss this one if you can; it rates only 1 star.

New Dimensions in Self-Care

The Eater's Guide to Tummy Tamers

Heartburn. Gas. Acid stomach. Ulcer pain. It reaches the point where you don't care how you spell relief—as long as you get it, and fast.

For the millions of Americans who suffer from the burning, aches and pains of digestive problems, there are hundreds of products that can bring relief. And they all do it essentially the same way—by neutralizing the stomach acid that's making your life miserable.

Everybody has stomach acid. You wouldn't be able to digest your food without it. Problems come up when it feels like it's digesting your stomach along with the food. With ulcers, that's just about the case. Since there's a break in the protective lining of the stomach, the acid is able to penetrate, causing the characteristic pain that usually accompanies ulcers.

But by far the most common use of antacids is for relief of *reflux esophagitis*—more commonly known as heartburn, acid indigestion or sour stomach. In these cases, the burning sensation doesn't usually take place in the stomach at all, but higher up, in the esophagus.

Normally, the stomach's contents are kept in the stomach and out of the esophagus by a special muscle, or sphincter, located between the two organs. But sometimes that muscle relaxes when it shouldn't, resulting in a reflux, or backing up, of the acidic juices. The lining of the esophagus is much more sensitive than the lining of the stomach, and it lets you know it by causing that uncomfortable burning sensation.

Antacids simply help neutralize the contents of the stomach so that the refluxed juices are no longer irritating. They don't neutralize all of the acid, but that really isn't necessary for the relief of pain.

Antacids have also been shown to increase esophageal sphincter muscle tone, and that action may add to their effectiveness in heartburn relief.

Actually, there's no doubt that antacids are truly effective. Ask any heartburn sufferer who's just swallowed an antacid.

Scientists have confirmed their usefulness, too. In one study, 33 heartburn sufferers were given either an antacid or a placebo (dummy pill) for a period of one month. Twenty-nine of the 33 correctly identified the antacid product, suggesting that the relief offered was not a placebo effect, say the researchers.

As for ulcers, antacids have been shown in clinical studies to not only relieve the symptoms but to actually promote healing as well. As one doctor said, "No acid, no ulcer"—and apparently he was right.

Still, all antacids are not created equal, even if the end result is the same. Here's why. Antacid products contain at least one of four primary neutralizing ingredients: sodium bicarbonate, calcium carbonate, magnesium hydroxide and/or aluminum hydroxide, all of which you'll find in a tablet or liquid base. For the most part, they pass through your system quietly, neutralizing the acid and putting a smile back on your face. But depending on how much you take, or what other underlying problems may also be present, there is the possibility of picking up some mild to possibly severe side effects along the way. A closer look at each of the four ingredients is needed to explain it all.

Sodium Bicarbonate

Sodium bicarbonate (Alka-Seltzer, Bromo Seltzer) is a potent, effective antacid and will relieve your symptoms of indigestion or heartburn. "Taken for occasional digestive discomfort (once a week or less) there's nothing to worry about. But it is definitely *not* recommended for more frequent use or for chronic conditions such as ulcers," says Nicola Giacona, Pharm.D., supervisor of the Drug Information Center at the University of Utah in Salt Lake City. Just a look at the name tells you why—*sodium* bicarbonate. "This is ordinary baking soda and it's loaded with sodium. Besides, it's completely soluble in the stomach and readily absorbed into the bloodstream, so it can lead to sodium overload and serious disturbances in the acid base balance of the body.

"Anyone on a salt-restricted diet (especially for high blood pressure) should forget products with sodium bicarbonate completely," adds Dr. Giacona. For example, a two-tablet dose of Alka-Seltzer contains 552 milligrams of sodium, enough to upset a salt-restricted diet.

The same is true if you're susceptible to fluid retention, since excessive sodium is usually involved with that problem, too. "Fortunately," says Dr. Giacona, "most brands have taken the sodium out of their products or reduced it drastically."

Calcium Carbonate

Calcium carbonate (Tums, Titrilac, Alka-2) is also an excellent acid neutralizer, besides being fast acting and inexpensive. While it is safe in small doses, regular or heavy use (more than six doses weekly) can lead to constipation.

"There is also concern that large amounts of calcium carbonate may cause acid rebound," Dr. Giacona told us. "That's when excessive acid is produced several hours after a dose of calcium antacid, setting up a possible vicious circle of acid secretion, antacid, acid, antacid and so forth."

In one study of 24 patients with chronic duodenal ulcers, taking four to eight grams of calcium carbonate induced excessive acid secretion 3 to 5½ hours later, whereas two to four tablespoons of aluminum hydroxide or four to eight grams of sodium bicarbonate did not (*Handbook of Nonprescription Drugs,* American Pharmaceutical Association, 1979).

Nevertheless, adds Charles B. Clayman, M.D., of Northwestern University Medical School in Chicago, "No one has shown that any of this has clinical bearing on the effectiveness of calcium antacids in the treatment of peptic ulcer."

Indeed, even the threat of kidney stone formation or hypercalcemia (excessive calcium in the blood) has been overplayed, Dr. Giacona says. "Our bodies are designed to compensate for variations of calcium intake. Unless a person has kidney disease, where the mechanisms break down and you can't eliminate the excess amount, those problems are uncommon. In fact, if you are taking a calcium supplement, it very likely is calcium carbonate—the same ingredient as the antacid, just without the flavorings that the antacid product has."

Magnesium Hydroxide

Magnesium hydroxide (Phillips Milk of Magnesia) is a little less potent in neutralizing capabilities than the two previous ingredients mentioned but is still very effective. Magnesium is rarely used as the only ingredient in a product, however, because of its well-known laxative effect. Most often it is used in combination with aluminum-containing antacids in order to counteract the constipation that commonly occurs with those products.

Magnesium-containing antacids pose a different threat to people with kidney disease, though. If excess magnesium can't be eliminated from your body, it may accumulate in your blood, causing a condition called hypermagnesemia. When that happens, your blood pressure drops, there's nausea, vomiting and ultimately, coma.

Aluminum Hydroxide

Aluminum hydroxide (AlternaGEL, Amphojel) is the weakest of the acid neutralizers and is rarely used as the sole active ingredient. Most often it is found in combination with magnesium products (Gelusil, Maalox, Mylanta), with sodium bicarbonate (Rolaids) or with calcium and magnesium (Tempo, Camalox).

Although constipation is the main side effect of aluminum-containing antacids, it is not the one that causes the greatest concern. Doctors used to think that aluminum passed through the body without being absorbed into the bloodstream. Now research has shown that not only is part of it absorbed but that some of it also binds with dietary phosphate and calcium, dragging them out of the body and possibly weakening the bones.

In one study, researchers decided to test the effects on phosphorus and calcium metabolism using small doses of aluminum-containing antacids. Seventeen men participated in the study and were given at least two tablespoons of antacid three times a day for a maximum of 36 days. The doctors also kept a check of each volunteer's dietary calcium and phosphorus intake.

The researchers found that even with small doses of aluminum-containing antacids, there was a significant increase in the amount of calcium and phosphorus excreted from the body (*American Journal of Clinical Nutrition,* July, 1982).

"Phosphorus depletion," says Herta Spencer, M.D., one of the researchers who conducted the study, "has been reported to stimulate bone resorption [loss], and this process would result in removal of both phosphorus and calcium from bone, thereby leading to an increase in urinary calcium. . . . The calcium loss induced by either increased bone resorption or decreased mineralization may eventually result in skeletal demineralization."

Indeed, says Dr. Spencer, "osteomalacia [adult rickets] has been reported in antacid-induced phosphorus depletion." What's more, this release of calcium from the bones can lead to or worsen osteoporosis, a bone-weakening disease.

On a more positive note, Dr. Spencer's study also showed that when calcium intake was approximately 800 milligrams per day (that's close to the Recommended Dietary Allowance, or RDA), these antacids did *not* result in a significant increase in calcium excretion, indicating that a diet high in calcium may reduce or counteract the antacid-induced bone resorption observed during low calcium intake.

Bursting Bubbles

You may have noticed that some products (Di-Gel, Maalox Plus) offer an additional ingredient called simethicone, specifically designed to reduce gas bubbles. There's been some question as to whether the claims are justified. The Food and Drug Administration says that simethicone is "safe and effective," but some doctors have their doubts. "The clinical data is scanty," says Dr. Giacona, "but there are some patients who swear by it. So, if it works for you, then use it."

There's no doubt, however, that antacids have made it easy to eliminate heartburn and acid indigestion. Maybe too easy. It's one thing to use them for an occasional attack of heartburn or indigestion and quite another to be popping tablets several times a day. "Any digestive symptoms that last more than two weeks should be checked out by a physician," advises Dr. Giacona, "since antacids may mask a more serious medical problem. For example, if your heartburn isn't immediately relieved with an antacid, the pain may be from angina, not indigestion—a symptom requiring prompt medical supervision."

Keep in mind that it's best to take antacids on a full stomach. On an empty stomach, antacids work only from 20 to 40 minutes. Taken one hour after eating, however, they continue to neutralize acid for up to three hours.

Also, antacids interact with certain antibiotics, heart medications and other drugs, so check with your doctor or pharmacist first.

And remember, it's still best to try to eliminate the cause of your digestive problem rather than accepting antacid gobbling as a way of life.

SOME HINTS FOR PREVENTING INDIGESTION

• Cut out caffeine-containing beverages. They increase acid production in the stomach.

• Avoid irritant foods, such as citrus juices, tomatoes and spicy foods.

• Avoid chocolate, alcohol, spearmint, peppermint and smoking. They lower esophageal sphincter pressure.

• Avoid fatty foods and large meals, which reduce gastric emptying.

• Wait at least three hours after eating before going to bed.

• Raise the head of your bed six to eight inches to improve stomach emptying.

• Avoid stooping or exercises that compress the stomach.

• Lose weight if necessary.

An Introduction to Self-Diagnosis

Diagnosis. It's one of those medical words that almost *smells* like a doctor's office. And, for most of us, it's something we'd think of attempting on ourselves about as soon as we'd consider performing an appendectomy. Yet you've probably diagnosed and treated yourself for minor medical ills dozens or even hundreds of times during your life.

You start feeling headachy, tired and feverish; you check your forehead and find it's hot, then—remembering your neighbor was recovering from the flu when you talked to him yesterday—you take your temperature and discover it's 100.2°F. So you take two aspirin and put yourself to bed. You've just diagnosed and treated a fever, probably caused by an influenza virus, using the same basic tools your doctor would use—a medical history (observing symptoms, recalling previous contacts), a physical exam (touching your forehead) and a medical test (taking your temperature).

Granted, you don't know exactly which bug you've got, but your doctor very likely wouldn't either, because the tests to pin it down precisely are expensive and time consuming, and wouldn't change his treatment at this stage anyway. In fact, says medical self-care pioneer Keith W. Sehnert, M.D., "People can become observers and treaters of disease *without* a firm diagnosis. Diagnosis is a professional, intellectual process practiced by physicians. But for most conditions, informed self-care and professional care are just about the same thing." Your doctor would put you to bed, based on the strong suspicion you had the flu, then check up on you the next morning—exactly what *you'd* do. In this case, at this point, a trip to see the doctor would be an expensive waste of time—for you, for the doctor and for the medical system as a whole.

As it turns out, in fact, most medical care doesn't involve a doctor at all, even among people who could readily afford one. Studies in the United States and Britain have shown that somewhere between 65 and 85 percent of all medical care is self-care. Which means a reasonable "working diagnosis" was made and a treatment plan followed. People aren't performing heart surgery on themselves, of course—most self-treated ills are probably fairly minor. But then, the vast majority of medical problems are minor, and relatively simple to diagnose and treat.

Dr. Sehnert calls it "the rule of 12": "Roughly once a month, or 12 times a year, most people get a headache, a cold, or some other self-limited condition. About 4 of those times, they'll seek professional medical help. But I believe more than half of those 4 times, people could take care of themselves just as well."

The statistics seem to bear him out: One British study found most doctors believe at least 25 percent of patient visits are for conditions people could just as well treat themselves. Donald Vickery, M.D., president of the Center for Consumer Health Education in Reston, Virginia, puts the figure much higher, at fully 70 percent. Believe it or not, most doctors would rather *not* hear all the details about your every ache and pain. In fact, in the British study, unnecessary patient visits for trivial complaints were the biggest single cause of frustration for the doctors surveyed.

There's another reason to consider relying on your own medical skills a little more often. Simon Rottenberg, Ph.D., a University of Massachusetts economics professor, has estimated that if just 2 percent of over-the-counter drug purchasers in the United States chose to go to a doctor rather than treat themselves, there would be a 62 percent increase in patients' office visits—292 million more doctor visits a year! "Even if we could afford to train the doctors to meet this demand, which we can't, and even if we could afford to wait for them to be trained, which we can't, we simply cannot afford to pay the bill for the visits," Dr. Vickery says.

In matters of medicine, the time for greater self-reliance is now.

But how do you become more medically self-reliant, in actual practice? By developing some of the same skills doctors themselves use. And first among them is a precise and observant eye. In fact, being an alert observer of your own symptoms is the first step in a medical self-care system that Dr. Sehnert teaches to corporations. Originally devised by Lawrence L. Weed, M.D., professor of medicine at the University of Vermont, the system is called SOAP. If it were widely put to use, Dr. Sehnert believes, unnecessary doctor visits would be cut in half.

The "S" in the system stands for "subjective," and it means "learning to describe your illness or injury and its history—the who, what, when and where of your symptoms," Dr. Sehnert explains. "It means not just 'I have a headache,' but 'I have a frontal headache that hurts only when I bend over and only on Thursdays.'"

Describing how he arrives at a diagnosis, Isadore Rosenfeld, M.D., has written: "A good doctor is a biological detective, using every clue that nature provides." So, like a detective, you need to teach yourself to discover and describe—*precisely*—every clue your body is handing you. If you have a pain, ask yourself where it is—exactly. What does it feel like—is it sharp or dull, steady or intermittent, stabbing or throbbing? How long does it last? And so on.

Two of the most important things to consider, Dr. Sehnert says, are *when* does the discomfort occur—"Ask yourself if the symptom follows any pattern: Does the backache always come after you've been sitting in a certain chair or car? Does the indigestion always follow your morning coffee? Is the symptom tied to any other symptoms?"—and does it seem to have a minor cause, one you can deal with yourself? If it's unusual, severe or persistent, don't hesitate to seek professional help.

Learning to ask yourself precise questions like this—to ask, in effect, the same questions a doctor would ask you—is a skill critical to competent self-care. A medical history is nothing more than a standardized series of questions, and "the medical history is without question the most important tool a doctor uses in arriving at a diagnosis in most cases," *Medical Self-Care* magazine coeditor David Sobel, M.D., told us.

Dr. Sehnert points out that by asking yourself precise questions, you become more attuned to your body—you learn to "speak body language," in fact. "And if we speak body language, the symptoms sometimes even tell us what to do for treatment." If you "tune in" to your sore throat and stuffy nose, for instance, you'll find your body saying, "My tissues are swollen! My throat is too dry! There's too much mucus in my nose!" It's also whispering suggestions—to humidify the air, drink fluids or use nose drops to temporarily reduce the swelling so you can breathe.

And, if you *do* end up visiting a doctor, you'll know more precisely how to describe your problem if you've paid attention to it. "Patients are lousy at explaining their symptoms," says Katherine Carson, M.D., a San Diego obstetrician/gynecologist and coauthor of *Take Charge of Your Body* (Blue Mountain Press, 1983). "They're too general, or they're unprepared, or they just don't really think about what exactly is bothering them."

That's a serious problem, because a doctor's diagnosis, to a large degree, depends on how you assess and describe your symptoms. (When you're caring for yourself, on the other hand, you have a natural advantage because you don't have to describe your symptoms to anyone but yourself, and you know better than anyone what feels right or wrong to your body.)

The "O" in the SOAP system stands for "objective." It means that the second step in medical self-care is an objective *measurement* of your symptoms. "Diarrhea ten times in one day is one thing; diarrhea four times a day is another," Dr. Sehnert told us.

Sometimes these measurements can be made with nothing more than a wristwatch (like taking a pulse), but more than likely they'll require the help of some basic medical equipment. Dr. Sehnert suggests including these items in a "family black bag" of self-help tools: a thermometer for taking temperatures; a stethoscope for checking heart sounds, congestion and breathing sounds; a sphygmomanometer for taking blood pressure; an otoscope for looking inside ears; and a high-intensity penlight for looking in the nose and throat and for transilluminating sinuses to check for congestion.

Exactly what tools you may need "will vary from person to person, family to family," Dr. Sobel says. "Most people wouldn't need an otoscope, unless they had family members with frequent ear infections, for instance." Nevertheless, being able to objectively measure symptoms is important. "There's nothing worse than a patient who calls and says with pinpoint inaccuracy, 'I ache all over,'" Dr. Sehnert says. "A phone call from a patient who knows how to take vital signs—pulse, respiration, temperature, blood pressure—and how to report relevant observations like inflamed throats or reddened eardrums is far more meaningful."

If your careful self-exam has narrowed your symptoms down to one simple, specific medical question—like the classic "was I sick this morning because I'm . . . pregnant?"—you may be able to get a simple answer with a medical self-test kit, one of the most remarkable medical tools now available to laypeople. At many drugstores you can now buy relatively inexpensive kits for testing for conditions ranging from pregnancy and urinary tract infections to internal bleeding and even vitamin C status. In their book *Do-It-Yourself Medical Testing* (Facts on File, 1983), Cathey Pinckney and Edward Pinckney, M.D., describe 160 such medical self-tests now available to the public.

Once you've made note of your symptoms and done what you can to objectively measure them, you need to take the third step—the "A" in SOAP—assessment. You "size up" the problem and figure out what to do. Is this your old familiar backache again—or are you also getting shooting pains in your leg? Is this "just" a cold, or has it hung on to the point where you've started to get worried?

Making a judgment call between what's a minor, self-treatable problem and one that merits a doctor's attention can sometimes be difficult. Fortunately, there are several good books to help you out. One is Dr. Vickery's *Take Care of Yourself: A Consumer's Guide to Medical Care*, with James F. Fries, M.D. (Addison-Wesley, 1977). Based on medical flowcharts he developed for physician's assistants at Fort Belvoir, Virginia, Dr. Vickery's book is laid out in graphic form, rather like a board game, with boxes and arrows leading you on a step-by-step course of action for your particular case. If you have a swollen gland in your neck, for instance, the chart leads you to the next question—"Is it associated with ear discomfort or sore throat?" If the swollen gland isn't in your neck, you move to a different question—"Is it located in the groin?"—and from there through a different series of actions leading either to self-care (with instructions) or a doctor's appointment.

Another good book is Dr. Sehnert's *The Family Doctor's Health Tips* (Meadowbrook Press, 1981). In a similar way, the book leads you to an informed assessment of your problem by providing information about what you need to know about the condition, what symptoms characterize it, what to check for, what self-treatment is best and "red flags" that signal the need to get professional help.

A new book, *Where Does It Hurt?* by Susan C. Pescar and Christine A. Nelson, M.D. (Facts on File, 1983), is organized a bit differently. When you don't feel well and you're trying to figure out what's wrong, you usually approach the problem in one of two ways, the authors reason. You may wonder if you have a specific health problem—"Could this be the flu?" "Do you suppose I've got appendicitis?"—and want to know if the symptoms you're experiencing really match those of that condition. Or you may be all too familiar with the symptoms, but have no idea what they mean—"I keep getting headaches, and they make me sick to my stomach. Do you suppose there's something really wrong?"

The book, as a result, is indexed both ways. you can look up your *symptom* and find out what diseases or conditions can cause it, or you can look up an *illness* to find what symptoms characterize it.

The final step in the process of self-diagnosis and self-treatment is to set up a treatment plan for yourself and stick to it. "Say to yourself, I'll try this home treatment for two days and if I'm not better by then, I'll go to a doctor," Dr. Sehnert says. If you're taking over-the-counter medications, pay attention to the treatment time limitation on the label. If you have any real doubts about how well your treatment plan is going, don't hesitate to err on the side of safety and see a doctor. But first, try trusting yourself a little. And remember, as Dr. Vickery says, when all is said and done, "*you* can do more for your health than your doctor can."

How to Have Healthy Breasts

Finding a lump in your breast can be frightening. Even when it's happily resolved with the diagnosis of "benign," the experience can leave you feeling vulnerable about this part of your body, wondering what you can do to avoid being a victim of chronic breast pain, or worse, being the 1 woman in 11 who gets breast cancer.

Knowing about your breasts—how they function and their disorders—is a good way to minimize that feeling of vulnerability.

Breasts are fat, honeycombed with milk-producing glands and ducts that respond to changes in body chemistry. The milk-producing cells lining the glands are controlled cyclically by three major female hormones—estrogen, progesterone and prolactin. In a woman of childbearing age, each month these cells are stimulated to grow and to accumulate fluids. This makes many women's breasts feel heavy, and sometimes painful and lumpy, three or four days before their period. When menstruation begins, this hormonal stimulation stops. In a healthy breast, the cell growth and fluids subside and the pain disappears.

In some women, though, premenstrual pain is severe or becomes a month-long problem. Why this happens is something researchers are still figuring out. It's most likely related to imbalances in hormone levels—too much estrogen or too little progesterone, says Robinson Baker, M.D., director of the Breast Clinic at Johns Hopkins Hospital, Baltimore. And it may be influenced by other body chemicals produced by stress or stimulated by certain foods.

Lumpy, painful breasts are one of many ailments that doctors place in the catchall category "fibrocystic disease."

"Most doctors will agree that lumpy, painful breasts are perfectly normal," says Susan M. Love, M.D., clinical instructor in surgery at Harvard Medical School. "Sixty percent of women have breasts painful enough to go to the doctor sometime during their lives. Not because they want relief from the pain but because they're worried that they have cancer. If you can reassure them that this is okay and that they do not need treatment, most are perfectly happy."

Other doctors *do* agree that painful, lumpy breasts are common. But, as we'll see later, they don't all agree that the condition is normal or necessarily healthy.

More severe forms of fibrocystic disease involve three separate types of breast conditions—fibrosis, the formation of cysts and changes in the cells lining the milk ducts, says Dr. Baker.

In fibrosis, the connective tissue that supports the milk duct grows and thickens into scar tissue, perhaps as a result of too much estrogen, Dr. Baker says.

In itself, fibrosis is not painful. But frequently it is accompanied by the formation of cysts. The milk ducts, blocked by tissue growth, are unable to drain properly and swell up into tender, fluid-filled sacs. Cysts can range in size from barely palpable to large enough to hold more than a quarter of a cup of water, and they can form in a week or two, Dr. Baker says. Small cysts often shrink on their own; larger cysts are often punctured and drained with a needle. If they recur several times in the same spot, they may be removed surgically.

Does having fibrocystic disease increase your risk of developing breast cancer? For years, doctors had been saying it does increase your risk by two to four times. Today, though, most say fibrocystic disease in itself does not lead to breast cancer—that is, cysts do not become cancerous.

Sometimes, though, some forms of this disease include overgrowth and abnormalities in the cells lining the milk ducts. This condition, known as proliferative, or hyperplastic disease, can develop into a malignancy, although only a small number do, Dr. Baker says. The only way to diagnose this condition is by tissue biopsy.

All women, whether they are at risk for cancer or not, should examine their breasts each month. For a woman with fibrocystic disease, though, the question is how to distinguish all those lumps and bumps from one that might actually be cancerous. This is where regular breast self-exams become important. The idea is to become so familiar with your breasts, lumps and all, that when you find something different or unusual, you recognize it for what it is and have it checked out. "Any discrete mass should be biopsied, regardless of a patient's age," Dr. Baker says. But there *are* ways to distinguish between benign and malignant lumps.

A cyst will be tender and move easily. It feels similar to an eyeball felt through an eyelid. A cancerous lump is often painless. It will seem to be anchored to the chest wall or to the breast tissue. Cysts can occur in both breasts simultaneously, but cancer usually occurs in one breast only, most often in the upper-right quarter nearest the shoulder.

Your own greatest risk factors for developing breast cancer are, unfortunately, things you cannot control. If your mother, sister or grandmother developed breast cancer, your own chances of getting it are two to three times greater than those of the general population. If the cancer developed prior to menopause or was in both breasts, the risk is even higher. If you've already had cancer in one breast, your chances of getting it in the other breast are fives times greater than if you'd never had cancer.

Breast cancer is unusual in women under age 30. Its incidence begins to rise in the early forties, but it's still relatively uncommon up to age 50. Most breast cancers are found in women aged 55 to 60.

There are ways, though, to decrease your odds, both for bothersome but benign breast ailments and for breast cancer. More and more prevention-minded health professionals are observing, and researchers are confirming, that breast disease is influenced by one factor we can do something about— our diet.

"I believe in taking a broad approach," says Phyllis Havens, a registered dietitian with the Holistic Center in South Portland, Maine, who counsels many women with breast tenderness and swelling and other premenstrual symptoms. "I recommend some major dietary changes and vitamin supplementation."

These include eliminating caffeine-containing foods and fat-rich dairy products, cutting back on red meats, sugars and fats, and adding safflower oil, fiber-rich vegetables and vitamins E and B complex.

The observation of Ms. Havens and others that this sort of diet relieves breast disease and problems with other estrogen-sensitive tissues like the uterus and ovaries is being confirmed, at least in part, by laboratory research.

John Minton, M.D., Ph.D., of the department of surgery, Ohio State University College of Medicine, Columbus, has found that substances contained in certain foods can aggravate breast symptoms. These substances produce biochemical signals that activate enzymes that promote fibrous tissue and cyst fluid development in women with fibrocystic disease.

"I know that most women can reverse lumpy, painful breasts completely with changes in their diet," he says.

Dr. Minton discovered that eliminating foods containing substances called methylxanthines (which include caffeine and are found in coffee, tea, cola and chocolate) was associated with the disappearance of breast cysts in most women within a few months.

But he also noted that some women who initially got much better on the diet later got worse.

"We discovered that when they stopped drinking coffee, they were somehow attracted to other foods that were giving them the same biochemical kick," Dr. Minton says. Although he is reluctant to say just what those foods are since his recent work has not yet been published, he does say that they include some dairy products, particularly cheese.

Christiane Northrup, M.D., a South Portland, Maine, gynecologist who refers some of her patients to the Holistic Center for nutritional counseling, prescribes 800 to 1,200 international units (I.U.) daily of vitamin E for her patients with fibrocystic disease. "I find it helps a great deal to relieve pain and swelling, especially when the symptoms occur because of rapidly changing hormone levels that come with menopause," she says.

Preliminary research by Robert London, M.D., director of reproductive medicine at North Charles General Hospital in Baltimore, suggests that vitamin E may be of value in treating breast cysts. In one study, 80 percent of the women responded to 600 I.U. of vitamin E daily for two months with decreased symptoms of pain.

His current work does not indicate that vitamin E lowers levels of estrogen or progesterone.

What about vitamin A? Can this apparent cancer inhibitor protect against breast disease? The answers aren't in yet, but there's a tremendous amount of interest in its possible use, says Marc Lippman, M.D., director of the National Institutes of Health Breast Cancer Division.

"The data from animal studies is quite encouraging," Dr. Lippman says. "Forms of vitamin A can prevent the action of some tumor promoters, there's no doubt about it." In tissue cultures, vitamin A prevents the proliferation, or uncontrolled growth, of breast tissue cells.

One of the most promising forms of vitamin A for breast cancer, based on work done by Richard Moon, Ph.D., is a retinoid called 4-hydoxyphenylretinamide, which was surprisingly effective in preventing breast tumors in mice exposed to carcinogens, says Frank Meyskens, M.D., associate professor in the department of medicine at the University of Arizona, Tucson. Researchers in Milan may soon be conducting a trial using this and other forms of vitamin A with women who have already had one breast cancer to see if it reduces the rate at which a second tumor appears.

Currently, in the United States, Maurice Black, M.D., of the Institute for Breast Disease of the New York Medical College, is using short-term high oral doses of both vitamins A and E in women who have had one breast cancer. This study arose as an offshoot of an ongoing investigation of the protective effect of specific cell-mediated immunity against the patient's own tumor. In the course of these studies patients were identified who lacked this immunity. It was those nonreactive patients who participated in the high-dose vitamin studies.

These women don't naturally show the kind of immune response associated with good survival rates, Dr. Black says. But with large doses of either A or E, 50 to 60 percent do show this immune response, and with both A and E 80 percent show the response, Dr. Black says. "We don't yet know if this induced response works as well as a spontaneous response. We haven't been following these women long enough to see if they have a reduced incidence of recurrent and/or second primary breast cancer." (Large doses of vitamin A shouldn't be taken without medical guidance.)

Selenium seems to have a protective effect. "The results of animal and human population studies continue to be encouraging that the risk of breast cancer does decline if selenium intakes are high," says Gerhard Schrauzer, Ph.D., professor of chemistry at the University of California at San Diego. In mice bred to carry a virus which puts them at high risk of developing breast cancer, those receiving extra selenium in their diet had an incidence of breast tumors that was 10 percent lower than those that received no additional selenium. "And there's increasing evidence that many human breast cancers have a similar viral influence," Dr. Schrauzer says. Mice fed a high-fat diet and exposed to cancer-causing chemicals also had fewer, slower-forming tumors with selenium supplementation.

"Human studies with selenium and breast cancer have yet to be done on a large scale, but ongoing studies in Finland and Australia with women with benign fibrocystic disease are showing that selenium supplementation does seem to have beneficial effects," Dr. Schrauzer says. This is a hopeful sign that this unpleasant condition will, in the future, become preventable and treatable by nutritional means. Foods high in selenium include seafoods, liver, kidneys, meat and some whole grains. Supplements of more than 200 micrograms shouldn't be taken.

Your best bet against both benign breast disease and breast cancer may be the same thing that helps protect against heart disease—a low-fat diet.

Population studies show a strong parallel between fat consumption and the incidence of breast cancer. Countries like Japan and Thailand, where low-fat diets are the rule, have only about one-quarter the number of breast cancer deaths as the United States, Denmark and the Netherlands, where people consume up to twice as much fat.

And in animal studies, the evidence is "overwhelming" that a high-fat diet enhances the development of breast tumors, says Clifford Welsch, Ph.D., a tumor biologist with a special interest in breast disease and a professor of anatomy at Michigan State University. Dr. Welsch and his colleagues are trying to figure out just what it is that links fat with breast disease.

"Our idea is that it promotes the secretion of hormones that stimulate the development of both hormone-responsive, normal and cancerous breast tissue," Dr. Welsch says. "It's my opinion that the evidence favors the theory that a high-fat diet increases the susceptibility of the breast tissue to hormone stimulus."

Forty percent of the calories in the average American diet come from fat, mostly in meat and dairy products like butter, cheese and milk. "I think we'd all do well to cut down by one-third to one half," Dr. Welsch says.

And it might be a good idea to replace some of that fat with high-fiber foods, such as whole grains and vegetables. Chronic constipation, something few people eating high-fiber diets experience, has been associated with breast disease.

Researchers at the University of California at San Francisco found that women with severe constipation (two or fewer bowel movements a week) were five times more likely to show signs of possible abnormal cell proliferation in fluids aspirated from their breasts than were women with normal bowel function.

"It may be that estrogen secreted by the liver is reabsorbed more readily by women with sluggish digestion," says Nicholas Petrakis, M.D., professor of preventive medicine at the University of California, San Francisco. "This could have a stimulating effect on breasts."

One other thing the doctors who treat breast disease frequently mention is stress. "Most of the women I see feel their symptoms are aggravated when they're upset or overworked," Ms. Havens says. One of Dr. Love's patients, a politician, suffers from breast pain only when she is campaigning.

"One's attitude, what we call the neuro-endocrine aspect of tumorigenesis, can markedly control the development of breast disease," Dr. Welsch says. "It affects the entire central nervous system and can really throw it out of whack."

What's a "good attitude" to have? It's not being so paranoid about getting cancer that you live in fear, but it's also not being negligent about checking your breasts for lumps each month—or taking other measures to reduce the risks, Dr. Welsch says.

A New Look
at Arthritis Drugs

The two faces of arthritis medications—the visages of help and harm—prompt pointed questions: Do the drugs' benefits outweigh their risks? Which ones are the most effective? Can they do anything more than simply suppress symptoms? Exactly how do they work?

Finding the answers means putting the sword to myths that are as old as the drugs themselves.

MYTH 1: Arthritis medications are simple substances with the simple function of killing pain • With over 100 enigmatic forms, arthritis itself isn't a simple disease, and the drugs used to treat it have matching complexity.

For one thing, antiarthritis agents aren't just painkillers, or analgesics, though they may contain some analgesic component. Usually, numbing the pain—and *only* numbing the pain—isn't entirely the point. Most serious forms of arthritis are basically an inflammation of tissue, most likely a joint. This means pain, all right, but also swelling, redness, heat, stiffness, even damage to the tissue. So the idea is to reverse the inflammation, reducing all its symptoms (including pain) in the process. Thus, like aspirin (the most-prescribed arthritis medication in America), most arthritis drugs are primarily anti-inflammatories. Through intricate processes that scientists are still arguing over, these substances try to cool inflamed joint tissue, the core symptom of the nation's number one crippling disease.

Arthritis experts have drawn clear distinctions between such anti-inflammatories and popular painkillers like Tylenol, Darvon, Demerol and others. James F. Fries, M.D., director of the Stanford University Arthritis Clinic and author of *Arthritis: A Comprehensive Guide* (Addison-Wesley), says that painkillers have little place in arthritis therapy.

"First," he says, "they don't do anything for the arthritis; they just cover it up. Second, they help defeat the pain mechanism that tells you when you are doing something that is injuring your body. . . . Third, the body adjusts to pain medicines, so they aren't very effective over the long term. This phenomenon is called tolerance and develops to some extent with all of the drugs we commonly use. Fourth, pain medicines can have major side effects."

But then side effects are some of the things that complicate arthritis drugs. They remind us that the drugs are complex blends of healing power and malevolent potential. Doctors don't even talk about selecting arthritis medications with few side effects, for the drugs average 30 or 40 possible adverse reactions apiece. Physicians speak of balancing the dosage that gives the most relief against the dosage that risks the most toxicity.

"Because of possible drug reactions, patients need to make sure they're taking the medication appropriately," says Paul H. Waytz, M.D., a Minneapolis rheumatologist. "And they need to alert their doctor to any problems. If they're this careful, side effects can be kept to a minimum and are usually reversible."

MYTH 2: Arthritis drugs are ultimate solutions to arthritis •
By now most arthritis sufferers know that drugs are not "magic bullets" that can kill arthritis forever. For, as arthritis experts keep insisting, the disease isn't curable like pneumonia or appendicitis. "With drugs we can control most signs and symptoms of arthritis," says Dr. Waytz. "We may even be able to force some forms of arthritis into remission. But we may not be able to completely eradicate the disease."

MYTH 3: An arthritis drug is equally effective for everyone with the same type of arthritis • Arthritics who believe this can end up scratching their heads when they compare notes with a fellow arthritis sufferer. Someone with rheumatoid arthritis (RA) may get relief with Motrin; another RA victim may not. Somebody with osteoarthritis may think Indocin's strong medicine; another afflicted with the same disease may say Indocin isn't strong enough. The wide variations in the way people respond to arthritis medications are a matter of scientific record.

"This lack of predictability in response is something that arthritics have to adjust to," says George Ehrlich, M.D., a rheumatologist and a visiting professor of medicine at New York University School of Medicine. "They have to be patient, for a doctor may need to switch them from one medication to another to find one that's effective."

And the medicinal options are many. There are over a hundred antiarthritis drugs around, many of them experimental and some of them as familiar to arthritics as table salt. They're a pharmaceutical spectrum that ranges from life-saving substance to medicinal reject. Here's a report card on the major categories.

Despite the recent appearance of upstart arthritis medications, the cheapest and most widely used antiarthritis preparation is still aspirin. Most rheumatologists recommend this ancient medicine (technically acetylsalicylic acid) as a first-line defense against arthritis—before trying the younger, high-tech concoctions. And even now it's frequently the yardstick by which other arthritis drugs are measured. Doctors prescribe it by the carload for several forms of arthritis, including osteoarthritis, juvenile arthritis and RA.

People who suffer from these types of arthritis, however, may be looking for different effects from aspirin. Some (like many osteoarthritis patients) may be after the mild analgesic component. Others (like those with RA) may need the potent anti-inflammatory response. But getting what you want means calibrating dosages.

Dr. Fries believes that the strictly analgesic effect of aspirin is maximum after two tablets (ten grains) and lasts about four hours. "In contrast," he says, "the anti-inflammatory activity requires high and sustained blood levels of the aspirin. A patient must take 12 to 24 tablets (five grains each) each day and the process must be continued for weeks to obtain the full effect." Such a regimen is standard therapy for RA sufferers and requires lots of medical supervision.

But often even a watchful physician can't avert what has frequently become headline news: aspirin's side effects. They range from mild to severe and happen in at least 30 percent of arthritics using the drug. Aspirin takers have had to contend with peptic ulcers, upset stomach, stomach bleeding, tinnitus (ringing in the ears), hearing loss, liver damage, even interference with the blood's ability to clot. On top of all that, aspirin is, next to penicillin, the drug most likely to cause an allergic reaction.

Many doctors argue, however, that you can avoid much of the gastrointestinal havoc by taking aspirin with food or using either coated aspirin or aspirin's almost identical twin, non-acetylated salicylate (which is not the same substance found in nonaspirin compounds like Tylenol).

The search for arthritis medications that are as effective as aspirin but less toxic led researchers to NSAIDs—nonsteroidal anti-inflammatory drugs. They're a handful of chemically diverse substances sporting brand names that arthritis victims have been hearing for years—Motrin, Indocin, Nalfon, Clinoril, Naprosyn, Butazolidin, Tolectin and others. They all have some analgesic potential, roughly as much anti-inflammatory power as aspirin and may therefore have the ability to prevent inflammatory damage. Whatever types of arthritis yield to aspirin yield also to NSAIDs.

But the similarities stop there. For one thing, these drugs, though more expensive than aspirin, generally require less pill taking to control RA. An RA sufferer, for example, may need to take only 2 Naprosyn tablets a day—but 15 aspirin. Doctors and patients both know that the fewer pills you must contend with, the more likely you are to stick with a dosage schedule.

And though NSAIDs cause most of the same side effects that aspirin does, the reactions are generally less severe. In fact, because of its safety record, one NSAID called ibuprofen (trade names: Motrin and Rufen) recently earned over-the-counter analgesic status as Nuprin and Advil.

Some doctors, however, caution that it's too early to hail NSAIDs as safer alternatives to aspirin. "Aspirin has been used for centuries," says Dr. Fries, "whereas experience with these new drugs is sufficiently limited that some side effects may not yet have been discovered."

Then there are those few NSAIDs that are giving the others a bad name. Oraflex and Zomax were removed from the market last year because they were associated with deaths.

And the serious side effects caused by phenylbutazone (Butazolidin) and indomethacin (Indocin) have raised grave doubts about their use.

An American Medical Association (AMA) guide to medications says that phenylbutazone can cause jaundice, hepatitis, blood in the urine, edema, rashes, gastrointestinal disturbances and—worst of all—bone marrow toxicity. Such toxicity can lead to aplastic anemia, a condition that's often fatal.

And Indocin's possible adverse reactions may be even more disturbing. It shares many of phenylbutazone's possible side effects (including bone marrow toxicity) and has some bizarre reactions of its own: eye disturbances, kidney trouble, confusion, coma, even behavioral problems. Perhaps most worrisome of all are the possible ulcerations of the esophagus, stomach and small intestine. Regarding this problem, the AMA says that perforation and hemorrhage (sometimes fatal) have been reported.

In the 1950s steroids took the medical world by storm, drawing enthusiastic praise from doctors and patients alike, capturing the unofficial titles of "wonder drug" and "miracle medicine." And, indeed, cortisone—the first of the steroid drugs—had actually enabled RA cripples to walk, run and even jump painlessly.

But then reality set in, says J.T. Scott, M.D., consulting physician at Charing Cross Hospital in London and author of *Arthritis and Rheumatism: The Facts* (Oxford University Press, 1980). It soon became clear, he says, that "the dosage of cortisone required to suppress the disease—and it did no more than that—produced also an alarming concatenation of toxic effects, ranging from the unsightly and hairy 'moon face' to perforating and bleeding gastric ulceration." And now, 30 years after the steroid debut, doctors are still wielding this medicinal two-edged sword—but more gingerly.

Corticosteroids are hormones manufactured by the adrenal glands. When the body gets an extra dose of the compounds (by injection of cortisone or prednisone, for example), inflammatory symptoms can be dampened down dramatically. NSAIDs or aspirin simply can't match this anti-inflammatory vigor.

Nowadays what doctors try to do in steroid therapy is

walk the thin line between this positive force and side effects like ulcers, skin disorders, bone disease and cataracts. And they do this by carefully controlling dosages and duration of treatment. Taking low-dose steroids for a short term or getting a single injection in a troublesome joint isn't likely to cause severe reactions in the properly selected patient. But long-term high-dose steroid treatment is practically guaranteed to cause health problems worse than arthritis itself.

"In certain cases of RA, steroids can actually be life-saving," says Sanford H. Roth, M.D., a Phoenix rheumatologist and the editor of *Handbook of Drug Therapy in Rheumatology* (Wright-PSG, 1984). "And low-dose steroids can be useful in select situations. But generally if we can achieve good results without steroids, we should not use them because of the many problems common to long-term hormonal therapy."

Remission-inducing drugs are chemically unrelated compounds that are the big guns of arthritis drug therapy—mighty medicines that can suppress symptoms for long periods, even bully the disease into remission. They originally were used to treat diseases other than arthritis, but now they're primarily for RA patients who've failed to respond to other drugs. And like all arthritis medications, they have their risks.

Gold salts (Solganal, Myochrysine and Ridaura) are probably the most popular remission-inducing compounds—among both rheumatologists and patients. They seem to work for about 75 percent of RA patients who try them, with some people achieving such deep remissions that neither doctor nor patient can detect the disease. But it can take weeks for therapy to start working. Once it does, however, the beneficial effects can last for months, long after the treatment is stopped.

How do these agents work? No one knows. They certainly exert an anti-inflammatory force, but scientists have yet to figure out why. How did anybody discover that the world's most precious metal has such therapeutic power? Accidentally. Years ago doctors thought RA was caused by tuberculosis (TB) germs, and since gold was being used to treat TB, they decided to try it out on RA patients. And it worked. It wasn't until later, though, that physicians learned—as they did with cortisone—that there was a physical price to pay for success.

Now we know that about 30 percent of those who receive

gold treatments will experience side effects—most of them mild but some of them life-threatening. Medical reports mention possible skin rashes, jaundice, mouth ulcers, kidney damage, blood disorders and aplastic anemia.

"Because of the potential problems, patients taking gold have to be carefully monitored," says Dr. Waytz. "They should have periodic urine tests and blood counts. And at the first sign of adverse reactions, the drug should be withdrawn."

All of which goes double for another remission-inducing drug called penicillamine. This by-product of the manufacture of penicillin has much in common with gold but has more potential for harm. Like gold, its workings are mysterious, long term and impressively effective (50 to 60 percent of patients will get some relief). But it has most of gold's possible side effects, plus a few more—gastrointestinal disturbances, autoimmune diseases, taste impairment, explosive vomiting and fatal bone marrow disruption. Some of these will occur in 40 to 50 percent of those who take the drug.

"Penicillamine," says Dr. Waytz, "should be administered in the lowest possible dose that will suppress the signs and symptoms of rheumatoid arthritis."

The antimalarial compounds, on the other hand, aren't nearly as toxic as gold or penicillamine—but then they're probably not as effective, either. They're derivatives of quinine, medications used around the world to combat malaria. Doctors don't know exactly how yet, but these agents (chloroquine and hydroxychloroquine) can offer relief to victims of several inflammatory diseases, including RA. It may take three to six months for the drugs to work, but the positive effects could last just as long.

Using the medications for such lengthy periods, though, is bound to cause some problems. Skin rashes, sores, gastrointestinal disturbances, hair blanching—these are the occasional and reversible penalties. A rare and possibly irreversible one is far more serious: blindness.

Weighing such risks against the benefits is the arthritis sufferer's lot—a serious business that requires a respect for medicinal power and a need for straight answers.

One arthritis sufferer, Christiaan Barnard, M.D., preeminent surgeon and author of *Christiaan Barnard's Program for Living with Arthritis* (Simon & Schuster, 1983), offers this advice: "Ask as many questions as you can: about length of time you will need to take the tablets offered, how they act, what their side effects are, what their dangers and potential benefits are. If the drug is newly developed, ask your doctor whether it genuinely offers something that other compounds already tried and tested on the market cannot provide. Play for safety, not spectacular overnight results. There are no miracles in medicine. Superb, marvelous treatments, but no miracles."

A Consumer's Guide to Laxatives

Laxatives are big business. Each year, in fact, we spend nearly $400 million on drugs that are supposed to bring us relief from that indelicate condition called constipation.

In a way, it's no wonder, because 41 million of us are plagued with constipation. And if you're one of the sufferers, you'll find more than 700 over-the-counter laxative products to choose from—a confusing situation, to say the least, especially since the active ingredients may vary from brand to brand.

Just because those drugs are available without a prescription, they're not necessarily safe. On the contrary, serious side effects are not uncommon with certain preparations.

The worst consequence is laxative abuse. That occurs when taking a laxative becomes so routine that it is virtually impossible to go without one. Year after year of laxative ingestion does not go unnoticed by your insides. According to Jacques Thiroloix, M.D., author of *Constipation: Its Causes and Cures* (St. Martin's Press), laxative sickness is almost inevitable when these products are taken for a long period of time. And the more toxic the laxative used, the sooner this condition appears.

"If laxatives are taken for a prolonged period, the chronic irritation will eventually alter the cells covering the internal wall of the colon [large intestine], exactly as if you'd sand-papered it every day," writes Dr. Thiroloix.

The results are devastating. The colon can no longer contract as it should, and normal intestinal muscle tone is shot. You're left with painful spasms—like colitis—where treatment leads, at best, to improvement but not cure. If you're smart you won't fall into that trap. There are safe ways to go about doing everything, and taking laxatives is no exception. Taken once in a while, laxatives are probably okay. But still, some are better than others. The best ones, according to the experts, help your own natural digestive processes along in the most harmless, gentle way. Here's how the major types of laxatives stack up.

Chemical Stimulants ● These are the strongest and most-abused laxatives. Chemical names to look for are senna (Senokot, Fletcher's Castoria), phenolphthalein (Ex-Lax, Correctol, Feen-a-Mint), cascara and danthron (Dorbane), bisacodyl (Dulcolax) and castor oil.

All of those chemicals work fast—usually in less than eight hours. Unfortunately, they may also produce painful cramps, diarrhea, dehydration and, when taken regularly, depletion of certain minerals from the body.

Doctors have advised against stimulant laxatives in general but have come down especially hard on the phenolphthalein ones. They're the most toxic of all the products that you could use for constipation, says Dr. Thiroloix. They act by irritating the colon wall. "The cells of the colon 'weep' under the assault, secreting a ropy, gluey liquid—mucus—which, mixing itself with the fecal mass, makes it more liquid."

The other chemical stimulants aren't much better. Bisacodyl can cause rectal burning. Senna and cascara are excreted in the breast milk of lactating women and can cause diarrhea in the infant. Danthron has been implicated in a case of hepatitis. And castor oil is potentially damaging to the lining of the small intestine.

Osmotic or Saline (Salt) Laxatives ● This type absorbs and pulls water into the feces for fast (two to six hours) and often liquid relief. They are also quite potent—almost as potent as the chemical stimulants, in fact. The most common ones include magnesium hydroxide (milk of magnesia), magnesium sulfate (Epsom salts) and sodium sulfate.

Besides the unpleasant effect of a liquid purge, these laxatives may pose a threat to patients with heart or kidney failure, due to excessive absorption of sodium or magnesium. What's more, the sodium laxatives can be harmful to those on a salt-restricted diet.

In this category, milk of magnesia is the mildest and could probably be tolerated if used infrequently.

Glycerin suppositories can also be classified here, too. They have no effect on the rest of the body, and they work in about 30 minutes. At worst, they can cause rectal irritation, but that's rare.

Lubricants ● These laxatives, such as liquid paraffin and mineral oil, act by coating the stool, allowing it easy passage.

Even though lubricants have been around for eons, doctors now feel that these agents should not be used in treating constipation. That's because, taken over a long period, mineral oil may deplete the body of all the fat-soluble vitamins (A, D, E, K). Besides, it can be messy, since it sometimes causes rectal leakage. It's even been suspected of causing an increased risk of gastrointestinal malignancies.

Stool Softeners ● These are like detergents. They promote the mixture of watery and fatty substances, which then penetrate the stool and soften it. The chemical involved is called DSS—dioctyl sodium sulfosuccinate (Colace). Although DSS does not interfere with the absorption of nutrients from the intestinal tract, it has been reported to enhance the absorption of mineral oil and should never be used along with it.

About the only time that stool softeners are really useful is after a heart attack or rectal surgery, when straining should be avoided.

Bulk-Forming Agents ● This type includes psyllium preparations (Metamucil, Effersyllium, Konsyl), polycarbophil (Mitrolan) and plantago (Siblin). They work by absorbing water and expanding. The added bulk stimulates contractions, while the absorbed water softens and fluffs up stools, making them easier to pass. These agents take a while to work—from one to three days. Their main function is to *prevent* rather than treat constipation.

Until recently, several of these products have been high in sodium, but manufacturers have since cut it back considerably. However, several of these preparations still contain as much sugar as they do the active ingredient. What's more, bulk formers must be taken with at least eight ounces of water (or other liquid) to prevent a possible blockage of the gastrointestinal tract. Even so, bulking agents are about the safest laxatives you can take, probably because they encourage your own system to do the work.

Keep in mind that unrefined bran, vegetable and fruit fibers and whole grains are nature's own bulk-forming agents. Put these in your daily diet and you'll probably have no need for the commercial bulk-forming products or any other laxatives.

How to Read Your Body Signs

You usually take a peek in the mirror to fix your hair, adjust your tie, put on your makeup or just generally check out how you look. But have you ever gazed in the mirror to see how you feel? It's not a bad idea, because that image mugging back at you contains evidence about the state of your health.

We've compiled a top-to-bottom checklist of visual clues, signs that you'd ordinarily ignore or overlook, which can tell you a lot about your present well-being and what the future might hold in store. So put vanity aside, slip into your birthday suit, face up to your full-length mirror, and give yourself a visual exam.

Your Eyes

Look yourself straight in the eyes. Are they bloodshot? Alcohol dilates the blood vessels in your eyes, so it may be a sign that you're overindulging. Have you been doing a lot of swimming lately? Chlorine can also make your eyes bloodshot.

If your eyes are chronically bloodshot, it's best to check with a doctor, because it could be a sign of infection or other disorder.

"If the blood vessels are *very* prominent, it could be an early sign of dry eyes or an infection," says Joseph M. Ortiz, M.D., an ophthalmologist from Bala Cynwyd, Pennsylvania. "For dry eyes, we generally recommend special eye drops called artificial tears. If they don't work in two or three days, however, you should consult a physician."

Now gently pull down on one lower eyelid. "The color inside should be pink to dark pink," Dr. Ortiz says. "In people who are severely anemic, it's quite white. That's because the color there reflects your level of hemoglobin. If you're a woman, it may be paler due to blood loss in menstruation. Just make sure you're getting enough iron in your diet."

Now look at the whites of your eyes, on the side nearest your nose. Are there small, raised bumps on the surface? Are they yellower than the surrounding area? If so, close your eyes almost all the way. Are the bumps at the midway level where your eyelids meet?

"Those bumps are called pingueculae," explains Dr. Ortiz. "They're evidence of sun damage. If you've spent a lot of time in the sun, you've probably been squinting. Pingueculae form where the sun gets through. They only become significant if they form on the edge of the cornea, the transparent part that covers the iris and pupil. Then they can tug on the cornea and hurt your vision. In addition, close attention must be paid, for any increase in pingueculae size could mean skin cancer.

"If you do have pingueculae, it's probably wise to avoid the sun, especially at midday," warns Dr. Ortiz. "Protect your eyes by wearing sunglasses that filter ultraviolet light or a hat with a brim that shades your eyes."

You probably know that puffy rings under your eyes can be caused by lack of sleep. "But," says Alan Gaby, M.D., of Baltimore, "they can also be a sign of edema (water retention) or a thyroid condition.

"If you're retaining fluid, your ankles may swell during the day due to the effects of gravity. But when you lie down at night the excess fluid will pool around your eyes where the skin is thinnest," adds Dr. Ortiz.

Do you have dark circles under your eyes? Dr. Gaby says

that may be a sign of allergy, but then again, it may mean nothing at all.

Your Face

Now stand back from the mirror just a little and observe the color of your face. Do you seem pale? "Pallor may be normal, healthy, and of the type much admired in a Victorian miss," says Joan Gomez, M.D., author of *A Dictionary of Symptoms* (Stein & Day, 1983). But "pallor arising in a formerly rosier face may be significant." Pallor can be a sign of anemia or kidney trouble, for example. But a yellow-white, papery complexion may just be a natural, normal consequence of old age, according to Dr. Gomez. However, "it is important to consult your doctor, as some conditions creating pallor may be serious," she cautions.

High color is usually associated with robust good health, but it can also be a sign of illness. For example, Dr. Gomez says that a ruddy complexion may be a sign of high blood pressure.

Does your skin look tough and almost corrugated? Does your smile have a permanent sag? Those are signs of solar elastosis, loss of skin elasticity caused by overexposure to the sun. And if that's not bad enough, severely sun-damaged skin can develop ugly brown patches (known as liver spots) or scaly gray patches (known as keratoses), which occasionally develop into cancer.

If the skin on your face and hands is tough and wrinkled but protected parts of your body are smooth and young looking, excess sun is most likely the problem. So take care now. Use sunscreens faithfully and avoid the sun's hottest onslaughts.

Your Mouth

Move close to the mirror again and open wide. Is the edge of the gum around your teeth bluish red or much brighter red than the adjacent gum tissue? "That's an indication of inflammation, infection or periodontal disease," points out Stephen Z. Wolner, D.D.S., of New York City. "Bone loss around the teeth begins with a simple case of gingivitis [gum inflammation]. That's the time for prevention, because bone loss eventually leads to tooth loss. See a dentist if you haven't seen one recently."

Next, look at your teeth where they meet the gums. Are there concave ridges there? "That's known as tooth erosion," explains Dr. Wolner, "and it can be aggravated by improper brushing. The tooth enamel is thinnest right at the gum line, so brushing back and forth with a hard-bristled toothbrush can wear a groove there." Changing to a soft-bristled brush and altering your style of brushing may arrest the process, but it might be necessary to resort to bonding to fill in the grooves.

While you've got yourself agape, check to see if you have any excessively worn tooth surfaces. "If the point of one tooth is worn down, or if your lower front teeth are very worn down, you may have a bite imbalance or you may be grinding your teeth," says Dr. Wolner. Your dentist can probably help you avoid doing further damage.

Your Back

Now grab a mirror, turn around and take a good look at your back. (You can close yur mouth now.) It's very important to keep an eye on all of those rarely glimpsed lumps, bumps and blemishes, because changes in them are the signs that point to skin cancer. "Melanoma, a particularly insidious and virulent form of skin cancer, often starts out from slightly raised skin lesions such as a mole or an age spot, and in the course of enlarging changes from a medium to a dark brown to a bluish or dark gray color," says Herbert Haessler, M.D., of Harvard Medical School, author of *Bodyworkbook* (Avon Books, 190). "But any skin blemish that changes in size, color or texture should be evaluated professionally without delay," he advises.

The only way to know if a mole has changed is to monitor it, making a note of its size and location. Changes in color, irregular borders or a rough, uneven surface are tip-offs to seek medical advice.

To check for poor posture, turn sideways to the mirror. Granted, it's probably not the most flattering perspective, but it's a useful one. "If your shoulders are very rounded or you seem very swaybacked, that can be a tip-off to future back problems," says Vicki Kalen, M.D., director of the Spinal Diseases and Trauma Clinic at Stanford University Medical Center. "Bad posture can fatigue muscles and make your back hurt."

Lawrence W. Friedmann, M.D., coauthor of *Freedom from Backaches* (Simon & Schuster), agrees. "A potbelly or swayback may be due to weak abdominal muscles, and that can cause back pain," he says. "And if one hip is higher than the other, it means one leg is longer than the other. That cause you to limp, stressing the muscles on one side." Uneven leg lengths can also cause scoliosis. Fortunately, it's easily corrected by inserting a lift into the shoe worn on the foot of the shorter leg.

"An extremely rounded upper back in the elderly can be a symptom of advanced osteoporosis," says Dr. Kalen. "But it doesn't happen overnight. Those patients have probably been calcium-deficient since early adulthood. The bones slowly get so weak they get squashed—it's called compression fracture. And surprisingly, there may be no pain. Doctors sometimes prescribe large doses of calcium, vitamin D, fluoride and estrogen to improve bone mass, but it doesn't always work." The best medicine for osteoporosis is prevention—in particular, making sure you get plenty of calcium.

Your Stomach and Hips

Are you overweight? If so, you've probably heard that you're at greater risk for certain disease. But recent research has discovered that it's not only *how* fat you are that matters, but *where* you're fat. Researchers at the Medical College of Wisconsin found that women who carry their extra fat around their waist are more likely to suffer from diabetes, high blood pressure, mental abnormalities and gallbladder disease than women who carry their extra bulk on their hips (*American Journal of Epidemiology,* January, 1984). Interestingly, an earlier study found no correlation between heavy thighs and diabetes *(Journal of Clinical Endocrinology,* vol. 54, no. 2, 1982).

A recent study of Swedish men, however, found that the bigger their waists in comparison to their hips, the higher the incidence of stroke and heart disease. The researchers conclude that the *distribution* of fat may be a better predictor of cardiovascular disease than the *amount* of fat (*British Medical Journal,* May 12, 1984).

Does your shape tell you you're at a higher risk for certain diseases? If so, do whatever is appropriate to reduce that risk, such as losing weight and cutting your salt, fat or sugar intake.

Your Legs and Feet

Now lower your gaze a bit and take a look at your feet. Do they point outward? Do your ankles appear tipped inward?

"If not treated, your feet may point out more and more over time, and your arches may become flattened. It's something that should be assessed professionally," says Richard H. Baerg, D.P.M., director of podiatric service for the Veterans Administration.

"The abnormal motion this condition causes can contribute to the early onset of osteoarthritis in the small joints of the foot. It might also cause excessive strain on the ligaments, leading to long-term problems such as joint inflammation. Treatment with an orthotic device [a shoe insert] can properly align the bones and alleviate the problem," he told us.

"If your knees and your feet *both* point outward, you may be headed for a hip problem," says Dr. Baerg. "It's common in older people. The muscles around the hip become less active, and there's natural swing to their gait. They seem to shuffle. It's a matter of allowing time to overtake your body. Engaging in a variety of muscle activities can prevent that from happening."

Wearing high heels for long hours over a long period of time can also cause leg problems. "If you look at your legs from the side, the line from the calf to the heel should have a natural curve, with an indentation above the heel. If yours is more of a straight line, your calf muscles may be shortened up," Dr. Baerg points out. "That condition can be reversed by exercise, stretching and gradually reducing the height of the heels you wear."

Well, that's it. You can put your clothes back on now. Just make sure to catch a glimpse of yourself in the mirror before you go out—you may have a hair out of place.

Say "No, Thank You," to These Folk Remedies

Grandma treated fevers with a compound from willow bark, drank fennel tea to relieve flatulence, held her breath to banish hiccups, and pushed chicken soup to combat the common cold. And you know what? She was right.

Evidence suggests that those and other folk remedies—steeped in tradition and thriving even under the cold gaze of some modern medicos—are right on target.

In fact, folk medicine has been hitting the mark with increasing numbers of medical professionals for two decades. Scientists have been scouring the globe for herbs that fight cancer and other ills—and have been finding them. Doctors have been logging clinical evidence of the powers of old-time cures. And medical academia has been finding more reasons than ever to take some of grandma's prescriptions seriously.

But closer scrutiny has also revealed that some folk therapies are worse than worthless. Like some treatments of modern medicine, the cures can be as bad as the disease. These are the remedies that give good folk medicine a bad name, for the best traditional therapies contradict neither human physiology nor horse sense. Here are some folk practices that fly in the face of both.

Whiskey

Maybe cowboys in TV westerns gulp down shots of whiskey when a poisonous snake bites their leg, but that's Hollywood. In real life this old remedy simply doesn't match medical evidence, which says that such a treatment could work more in favor of the snake than the victim.

"Whiskey dilates your blood vessels," says Howard Posner, M.D., medical director of the Center for Preventive Medicine and Dentistry in Bala Cynwyd, Pennsylvania. "And when that happens, the venom can get into the bloodstream much faster. There's no question: Whiskey and snakebite is a potentially dangerous combination."

Snow

Perhaps the idea of rubbing snow on frostbitten skin came from Hollywood, too—or maybe some chuckleheaded woodsman. Common sense says it's wrong, and in light of the physiological facts, it stands convicted as a dangerous notion. "It's definitely the wrong thing to do," says Daniel P. Marshall, M.D., a Memphis physician and coauthor of *Staying Healthy without Medicine* (Nelson-Hall, 1983). "The snow would only cause more chilling of the skin and more constricting of blood vessels—an open invitation to permanent tissue damage. What's required is slow and gentle warming of the affected area by immersion in lukewarm water."

Sassafras

This ancient herb has a reputation as a stimulant, an antispasmodic (muscle relaxant), a sudorific (sweat producer), a treatment for rheumatism, skin diseases, typhus and who knows what. And oh, how tasty its tea. But its real character belies all its pleasant associations.

Sassafras contains safrole, an oil once used in root beer and similar beverages, and safrole has been shown to cause cancer in laboratory rats and mice. That was enough to prompt the Food and Drug Administration (FDA) to ban both sassafras and safrole as flavors or food additives.

"No one really knows just how harmful sassafras is to human beings," says Varro E. Tyler, Ph.D., an herb expert from Purdue University and the author of *The Honest Herbal* (George F. Stickley Co., 1982). "But it has been estimated that one cup of strong sassafras tea could contain as much as 200 milligrams of safrole, more than four times the minimal amount believed to be hazardous to man if consumed on a regular basis."

Comfrey

People swear that this herb is one of the best external medicines Mother Nature ever devised. They apply it as poultice or paste to boils, bruises, skin ulcers or wounds—and report rapid healing. And available evidence seems to back them up, for scientists have shown that comfrey contains allantoin, an agent that promotes cell proliferation and therefore healing.

But *drinking* comfrey—as tea—is another matter. Both the root and leaves of comfrey have caused cancer in rats, even when the herb was only a tiny part of their diet.

One of the nation's foremost experts in drugs derived from plants, Ara Der Marderosian, Ph.D., of the Philadelphia College of Pharmacy and Science, says, "I would not recommend that comfrey tea be consumed at all, even in small doses."

Pennyroyal

The name actually refers to two dissimilar herbs in the Mint family, one American and the other European. Both are supposed to help alleviate intestinal gas, stimulate the senses, produce sweating, even induce abortion. But if they do have therapeutic power, it's mixed with deadly potential.

"American pennyroyal contains up to 2 percent of a volatile oil," Dr. Tyler says, "and European pennyroyal up to 1 percent of an even more disagreeable-smelling volatile oil. Both oils consist of 85 to 92 percent pulegone—an organic chemical—and are therefore quite toxic, causing severe liver damage even in relatively small amounts."

Indeed, there have already been at least two deaths associated with the herb, one of them attributed to a mere one-ounce dose of pennyroyal oil. Which is a reminder of the law that every good herbalist embraces: The extracted oils of medicinal plants are not to be trifled with.

Cobwebs

Maybe your uncle John said that the best bandage for an open wound is a cobweb, and maybe he heard it firsthand from his grandfather, but that doesn't mean the treatment works. It doesn't. The elementary medical fact is that it just makes matters worse.

"Putting cobwebs on a wound is just asking for infection," says Dr. Marshall. "There's no telling what bacteria you'd be applying to the affected area. If we know anything about open wounds, it's that they must be kept clean to heal properly."

Ice-Water Baths

To some people, it makes perfect sense to give a heat-stroke victim an ice-water bath. After all, heatstroke is caused by prolonged exposure to heat. Your temperature rises, your pulse speeds up, your skin gets dry and hot. And a nice dip in icy H_2O could put the fire out. Sure—and kill you in the process.

We now know that such a sudden change in temperature can be more than a body can stand. "It's a dangerous technique," Dr. Posner says. "It may be too much of a shock to the patient's heart. The correct treatment for heatstroke is an immediate trip to the hospital."

Mistletoe

Deck the halls with it, hang it on the Christmas tree, use it as an excuse for holiday smooching, but don't even think of making tea with it. Mistletoe is poisonous. Not just the berries—your mother warned you about those—but the leaves as well.

Legend has it that American mistletoe stimulates the smooth muscles, raising blood pressure and triggering uterine and intestinal contractions. The European breed is supposed to have precisely the opposite effect. But animal studies show that the active ingredients in both types bring on similar calamities—decreased blood pressure, slowing and weakening of heartbeat and constriction of blood vessels.

It's little wonder then that both varieties showed up on the FDA's official list of unsafe herbs. And apparently most experts are in full agreement.

Camphor

This remedy is as old as the hills and almost as permanent. People have used it for everything from chest colds to bug bites and probably always will. But in the tradition lurks danger.

According to a national poison control center, camphor is a known toxin in humans. As little as one teaspoon of camphorated oil—a liquid form of camphor and linseed oil—can be toxic to a baby.

Indeed, there are reports of at least 12 people dying because of camphor poisoning. The FDA has taken camphorated oil off the market, and a non-FDA report says that over-the-counter products with more than 2.5 percent camphor are dangerous.

Calamus

This herb (sometimes called sweet flag) was known in biblical times and is still recommended today by herbal enthusiasts who should know better. Drink calamus tea for fevers and dyspepsia, they say. Chew it for good digestion and a clear voice. Pulverize it and use it to spice up your cooking. Only trouble is, calamus causes tumors and other abnormalities in laboratory rats.

It has therefore made the FDA unsafe herb list, and its long-term use has been condemned by informed herbal experts. According to Dr. Tyler, "the utilization of calamus as a home remedy or of calamus-containing products for any purpose is no longer rational."

Manure

Manure? Right. As repulsive as it sounds, a bona fide folk palliative for bee stings and bug bites is to dab on some manure. True, a cool, damp dressing can soothe itchy skin, and maybe manure does the trick. But the folks who originally reached for animal droppings reached a terrible conclusion, for putting manure on a bite or sting risks infection—or worse.

"Tetanus spores live in manure," says Dr. Posner. "And so using manure is dangerous. It's an old folk remedy that has actually killed many people. I suggest honey, lemon juice or clay as a remedy for bee stings and bug bites."

Coltsfoot

This is the legendary antidote for coughs and bronchial congestion. No doubt Grandma concocted a fine coltsfoot tea or made some coltsfoot cough drops or syrups. And perhaps the remedy did all the soothing it was supposed to do. But recent research has uncovered another side to the herb.

Some investigators in Japan have found that the plant's

dried flowers caused liver tumors in rats. And the rest of the herb has proved suspect as well.

"People suffering from throat irritations can no longer consider coltsfoot preparations appropriate therapy," says Dr. Tyler. "Neither the flowers nor the leaves can safely be used for medicinal purposes."

But, he says, there are other herbs that can soothe your throat. Slippery elm bark or marshmallow root, for instance. And like most good folk remedies, they offer you healing alternatives you can live with.

The Male Version of Breast Examination

"Testicular cancer is not a very common cancer among men. It occurs much less frequently than breast cancer in women. But for the men who get it, the statistics don't matter," says Richard D. Williams, M.D., a specialist in urological cancers.

As chief of urological oncology at the University of California Medical School in San Francisco, Dr. Williams treats men who get testicular cancer. He's one of a growing number of experts who believe all men should perform a monthly three-minute exam to check for lumps on their testicles. Lumps are one of the early signs of cancer there.

If caught early, testicular cancer is one of the most curable of cancers, says the American Cancer Society. If not caught early, it is one of the most deadly, because it spreads quickly to other parts of the body. It is a rare disease, accounting for only 1 percent of cancer in all males and only 3 percent of cancers of the male urogenital organs.

Testicular cancer is principally a young man's disease. It occurs mostly in men aged 18 to 40. But Dr. Williams says he's treated testicular cancer in boys under 18 and men over 40, too. There's simply a much lower incidence in those age groups. For that reason, Dr. Williams thinks all men should perform the self-exam from puberty on.

Other men who are at much higher risk for testicular cancer are those whose testicles didn't descend properly into the scrotal sac shortly after birth. The condition can be easily corrected in male infants, and the American Cancer Society recommends that parents have male babies checked for this reason.

We asked Dr. Williams why the testicular-cancer self-exam isn't more widely known among men. "I think we're just coming out of an era when touching yourself was not talked about. Now there's an explosion in learning about your own body," he says.

The American Cancer Society says the first sign of testicular cancer is usually a slight enlargemment of one of the testicles and a change in its consistency. Pain may be absent, but often there is a dull ache in the lower abdomen or groin, together with a sensation of dragging and heaviness.

The best time to perform the self-exam is after a warm shower or bath, when the scotal skin is most relaxed, says the American Cancer Society. Roll each testicle gently between the thumb and fingers of both hands. If you find any hard lumps or nodules, you should see a doctor. Dr. Williams says that men can remind themselves to do the self-exam by performing it on a set date, perhaps the first of each month.

When a lump is found, the affected testicle must be surgically removed—that's the only way to check for malignancy. However, malignancies are almost always confined to one testicle. The remaining testicle is perfectly capable of maintaining sexual fertility. Gel-filled implants can be inserted where the testicle was removed, for men who wish it.

Though the risk of testicular cancer is low, says Dr. Williams, the self-exam is worth it. "There are only certain parts of the body we can actually feel for cancer. So I tell men, 'Why not do it?'"

Environmental Health Updates

Is Your Pet Contagious?

"Anyone who hates children and dogs can't be all bad," W.C. Fields once remarked acidly. But the comic's view has never gained much of a popular foothold. Today the households of America put the Ark to shame, with something like 90 *million* dogs and cats (not to mention parakeets, gerbils, snakes, fish, monkeys and all the rest) sharing living quarters with their human companions. Pets—and children—are a bother, but how much poorer life would be without them!

Still, there *is* a price. Animals, like humans, play host to their fair share of disease-causing microorganisms, and some of these (about 40 in all) can be passed from household pets to their masters. Called zoonoses, these pet-borne diseases usually use animal bodies as way stations in their complex life cycles, but have learned to make the crossing to human bodies if one is handy. Some of these diseases are rather mild and self-limited, like cat scratch fever. Others are potentially more serious, like toxoplasmosis, which can cause birth defects if a woman contracts the disease during pregnancy.

The bad news is that most animals who are carrying around an infectious bug don't look sick. Many show no symptoms at all. And, because it's so difficult to track down the source of an illness, and because humans who pick up zoonoses often have only the vaguest of symptoms, researchers believe pet-borne diseases spread to humans far more often than is actually reported.

Children are at special risk. They love to put their hands and fingers in their mouth, giving bacteria a free ride to a new home. Kids are also more susceptible to illness because they cary fewer antibodies than adults do (having been exposed to fewer diseases in their short lifetimes). The same is true of baby animals. That's why kittens and puppies are more likely to be disease carriers than adult cats and dogs.

The good news is that pet-borne diseases are actually fairly rare, no matter how you count the numbers. "People are always quick to blame animals, but the fact is people acquire most diseases from other people," says Dorothy N. Holmes, D.V.M., Ph.D., a senior research associate at the New York State College of Veterinary Medicine at Cornell University. Usually, she adds picking up a pet-borne disease requires very close contact with animals or their excretions, so it can nearly always be avoided with a little common sense, cleanliness and regular pet vaccinations. Taking care of your pet's health is taking care of your own.

Surely the most famous, and scariest, pet-borne disease is rabies, a virus of the brain and nervous system. If you're bitten by a rabid animal and not inoculated, once the clinical symptoms appear it's almost invariably too late to save your life. There are only two cases on record of humans recovering from rabies (one, surprisingly enough, a six-year old boy).

Fortunately, human rabies is extremely rare—there are only one or two cases in the United States each year, mostly from wild-animal bites. But because the virus is so dangerous, about 30,000 people end up getting postbite rabies shots as a precaution each year. They're uncomfortable, but worth it.

Much less dramatic but far more common than rabies, salmonellosis is caused by group of bacteria that usually make their way into human bodies through contaminated food. But you can also pick them up from dogs, frogs, aquarium snails, turtles and the feces of pet chicks. Salmonella poisoning from pet turtles was so common in the mid-1960s—causing an estimated 280,000 cases yearly—that the Food and Drug Administration (FDA) banned their sale in 1975. Dogs carrying the bacteria usually show no symptoms but shed the bacteria in their feces.

If you pick up salmonella from your pet, it usually results in fever, vomiting, diarrhea, exhaustion and occasionally—in the very young, very old or sick—even death. Cleanliness is the best way to avoid it. Wash your hands after handling aquarium pets, keep kids away from dog droppings, and don't keep pet birds in rooms where food is prepared, because the bacteria are fond of growing in food kept at room temperature.

One of the most common transmissible pet diseases Seattle vet George Thue, D.V.M., sees in his practice is roundworms. "Some adult dogs and cats and most puppies carry roundworms, and the eggs are excreted in the feces," Dr. Thue says. "Youngsters, especially, are apt to pick up the eggs after playing with animals or their feces and then putting their hands in their mouths." Once swallowed, the eggs may hatch out and the larvae travel to the liver, muscles, eyes or central nervous system. The infection may cause a flu-like illness with fever, cough, loss of appetite, weakness and lung congestion, or sometimes even seizure disorders and myocarditis, an inflammation of the walls of the heart.

All puppies and adult animals should be examined for roundworms, Dr. Thue advises. And parents should keep young children away from areas soiled with dog feces. Sandboxes should be covered when not in use.

Cat scratch fever, Dr. Holmes says, "has been an enigma for a long time," because sometimes it's associated with a cat scratch and sometimes it's not. Ten percent of patients report no contact with a cat at all. But recently, researchers at the Armed Forces Institute of Pathology in Washington, D.C., reported they'd found what they believe is the guilty party, a kind of bacteria that may or may not enter the body riding a cat claw. If you do pick up this bug, it's likely to cause a persistent high fever, loss of appetite, weakness and (the most characteristic sign) swollen lymph nodes. It's fairly mild and usually goes away by itself.

If the scratches are really deep, you may contract a rare but more serious infection from the *Pasteurella multocida* bacterium. Pasteurella lives in the mouths of about half the dogs in the United States and almost all cats. It can cause localized tissue destruction and sometimes bone infection and blood poisoning. Doctors recommend treatment with penicillin, which effectively knocks off the bug, after any deep scratch or bite.

Stuart Copperman, M.D., a suburban New York pediatrician, recently reported a surprising discovery: In families plagued by repeated strep throat infections, 40 percent of the family pets turned out to be harboring active strep organisms. Most of these dogs, cats and birds showed no symptoms of strep themselves, Dr. Copperman found, but in every case, antibiotic treatment of the infected animal put a stop to persistent strep throat in the children. If strep throat is dogging your family, have the family pet checked, he suggests. And keep kids from kissing, licking or exchanging food by mouth with their pets.

Heartworm is a deadly disease in dogs. Carried by mosquitoes, these parasites migrate to the dog's heart and major blood vessels, where they can grow up to a foot long. Infected dogs tire easily and may suffer from labored breathing, frequent coughing and general sluggishness. If untreated, they can die. When humans pick up the parasite through a mosquito bite, the effects are so minor most people don't even notice them. The trouble is, the parasites can migrate to the lungs, producing a coinsized lesion that looks just like cancer on x-rays. The needless surgery that may result is the main risk of heartworms to humans.

By contrast, the cat-borne disease toxoplasmosis can cause serious harm to a developing fetus if a woman picks it up during her pregnancy. The disease is caused by an intestinal parasite called *Toxoplasma gondii,* which humans can contract from two main sources: raw or undercooked meat, and cats. Cats are the only animals that carry the adult parasites, having usually gotten the infection from raw meat. Once a cat becomes a carrier, it passes off the parasite's eggs in feces for two or three weeks, then becomes immune and rarely if ever sheds them again. However, infected cat feces can still infect humans for as long as 18 months.

When humans get the parasite into their system, they usually feel no ill effects, then develop antibodies and become immune. Ingesting a really large number of eggs can cause illnesses ranging from something resembling a mild cold to painful lymph nodes, fever or eye infections. But if toxoplasma infects a pregnant woman who is not immune, it may sometimes cross the placenta and cause a spontaneous abortion, or cause blindness, cleft palate, mental retardation or neurological disorders. On the other hand, the infected mother may give birth to a normal, healthy (and lucky) baby.

"Cats have gotten a lot of bad press because of toxoplasmosis, but really, you're much more likely to pick up the parasite from raw or undercooked meat," Dr. Holmes explains. "One study at a French maternity clinic showed that French women, who like to eat undercooked, pink lamb, had a greater tendency to develop toxoplasmosis during pregnancy than Vietnamese women, who didn't eat as much pink meat."

From whatever source, toxoplasmosis in pregnancy is quite rare — only about 1 in 3,000 pregnancies is believed to be complicated by the disease, and not all of these result in birth defects. Still, it's important to do everything you can to protect against it. Pregnant women should never empty the cat's litter box (get someone else in the household to do it daily), and wear gloves when gardening, especially in places where cats may have defecated. Cats shouldn't be fed raw or undercooked meat, and all meat for human use should be cooked thoroughly. If you're still concerned, tests are available to check for immunity — in humans or in cats.

Swimming in a farm pond or playing in a puddle are two great joys of childhood. Unfortunately, they're not without a certain risk. Humans can contract leptospirosis through direct contact with urine from an infected animal, or water contaminated with it. It's usually acquired from pigs or cattle, but dogs can also carry the organisms, which may cause fever, acute headaches, chills and sometimes nausea and vomiting. It's relatively rare — in 1982, 61 cases were reported in the British Isles — but can sometimes be severe (four victims died).

It's a good idea to keep animals away from swimming pools, and keep kids from playing in puddles that may have been contaminated with dog urine.

A lung infection called psittacosis can be passed to humans through birds — parakeets, pigeons, chickens and parrots — usually through inhalation of cage dust. "There's been an increase in this disease in the last few years," Dr. Holmes says. "Even though there are regulations about keeping birds in quarantine

before they're brought into the country, some always slip through."
Infected birds look droopy, have ruffled feathers and eat poorly;
infected bird owners suffer chills and headaches, loss of appetite,
fever and a hacking cough. Fortunately, psittacosis can be
diagnosed through a blood test and treated with tetracycline.

Dogs, cats and other animals can also play unwitting host
to some rather unpleasant guests—things like fleas and ticks.
Usually flea bites just itch (about half the human race is
allergic to them), but sometimes they can transmit diseases
like tapeworm, a plaguelike fever called tularemia, and even
plague itself. It's notoriously difficult to get rid of fleas once
they've established themselves in your house, but it's worth it.

Ticks can carry Rocky Mountain spotted fever, an infectious disease that's usually fairly mild but can occasionally be
fatal. Its characteristic sign is a rash on the wrists and ankles,
as well as fever, headache, muscle pain and mental derangement.

In short, there *are* some risks to sharing your life with an
animal, but your pet's love, loyalty and warm tongue are
probably well worth the trouble. A few simple precautions are
in order, however. The most important considerations, Dr.
Holmes says, are to keep your animals vaccinated and see that
they get regular veterinary care. It's also best to avoid stray or
sick animals, and to buy pets from reputable sources.

The next most important factor is cleanliness. Don't lick
or kiss your pets, keep their dishes separate from yours, and
keep youngsters away from their excretions. To keep litter
boxes clean, Dr. Thue suggests putting only a very small
amount of cat litter in the box, then emptying it completely
each day. By keeping your animal clean and vaccinated, you'll
help keep illness out of BOTH your lives.

Light Up Your Health

One autumn, as the days grew shorter and the nights
longer, Weldon Ellis decided to change the lighting scheme in
the study of his home in Nashville, Tennessee. The 74-year-old
retired architect and writer had found himself facing yet another
bout with the "end-of-the-year doldrums," as he put it, when

he happened to read that very bright indoor lighting can help susceptible people banish their wintertime blues.

As one who believes in taking his health into his own hands (he works out on a mini-trampoline and has taken supplements for years), Ellis set about making his study brighter. He replaced the standard 75-watt bulb in his desk lamp with a broad-spectrum "grow light." Then he mounted a track on the ceiling and installed a pair of 150-watt floodlights, one over each of his shoulders.

"So many people complain about a lack of pep in the winter," Ellis recently told us. "And the reason might be that we've been underlighting ourselves. It's a seat-of-the-pants sort of thing, but when I put the lights in, I found that I could work longer and later than before. You might say," he adds with a chuckle, "that I 'saw the light.'"

In essence, Ellis created in his study the lighting conditions of a spring day. Whether or not his floodlights really did give him a case of spring fever in January, we can't say. But, in spirit, he was rediscovering a phenomenon that many psychiatrists and endocrinologists have recognized in recent years: Light can have a very complex effet on the body and it does much more than enable our eyes to see.

Although the process isn't entirely understood, it's believed that light enters the eye, travels to the brain and stimulates the pineal gland. Depending on whether light is coming in or not, the pineal gland either suppresses or releases a hormone called melatonin. This hormone induces sleep, raises the level of serotonin (a neurotransmitter that carries messages through the nervous system) and determines the release of still more body-regulating hormones. In short, light seems to have tremendous impact on our health and behavior.

Two researchers in particular have made great contributions to our knowledge of light and health in the past decade. One is Richard Wurtman, Ph.D., of the Massachusetts Institute of Technology. He has maintained for years that most of us do not receive enough of the right kind of light for optimal health. The artificial lights that we typically use indoors provide only about one-tenth of the light available outside under a shade tree on a sunny day, he says. And artificial light, at best, isn't as beneficial as sunlight. Dr. Wurtman has shown that light, among other things, helps determine female ovulation, affects the ability of older people to absorb calcium and can be used to treat jaundice among newborns.

Another leader in light research has been John Ott, who learned about the effects of light on plants while he was a time-lapse photographer for Walt Disney studios. A nonscientist, he has written two influential books on light (the latest is *Light, Radiation and You,* Devin-Adair, 1982) and believes that most artificial light lacks essential wavelengths in much the same way that refined flour lacks certain vitamins and minerals. He claims that certain cells in the body can't function without those parts of the spectrum, and that most indoor lighting promotes illness, including cancer.

Other researchers have been building on the work of Ott and Dr. Wurtman. Some of the most promising breakthroughs have been made in the treatment of depression.

Light specialists now know that certain types of depression arrive in the winter and vanish in the spring. A surprisingly large number of people lapse into a wintertime funk when Daylight Saving Time ends. As one researcher put it, "Hibernation is not unknown among the human species."

"Most people say that they slow down a little in the winter," says Thomas Wehr, M.D., of the National Institute of Mental Health. "They sleep more, they gain a little weight. The number of people who have an extreme problem is larger than we thought at first. These are people who know that something is wrong, but they've never known what to call it."

In some cases, a mild funk turns into a serious mental illness. "The people we're seeing right now have severe symptoms," Dr. Wehr told us. "They're almost incapacitated by it. They stop cooking meals, they don't see their friends. They are experiencing a great deal of stress and they may even become suicidal."

Dr. Wehr and colleague Norman Rosenthal, M.D., recently treated a 63-year-old manic-depressive man whose depressive periods almost always began in midsummer and peaked around year's end. While depressed, he withdrew and became self-critical and anxious. He complained of fatigue and was afraid to go to work. Attempts to treat him with drugs were abandoned due to side effects.

With this pattern in mind, the researchers decided to bring the man out of his depression by doing something remarkably simple: They created the conditions of a spring day. During the first week of December, several weeks before the patient's depression was scheduled to end, the doctors woke him at 6 A.M. and exposed him to very bright artificial light—about ten times as bright as customary indoor light—for three hours. Then at 4 P.M. they exposed him to the same type of light for another three hours. In effect, they were lengthening his days. The treatment lasted ten days.

Within about four days, the man began to emerge from his depressive cocoon. In his own opinion, he felt much better. And the nurses who observed him thought so, too. The researchers came away from the experiment believing that humans, like bears and migratory birds and most of what used to be called the animal kingdom, have seasonal rhythms. Although the beneficial effect ended four days after the treatment ended, the researchers had established that strong artificial light can have as great an effect on mental health as does natural sunlight (*American Journal of Psychiatry,* November, 1982).

Strong artificial light can also have an effect on people who suffer from depression year-round. Daniel Kripke, M.D., of the University of California, San Diego, believes that depression may occur when the body's circadian rhythm goes awry and the body's inner clock runs too fast or too slow.

He thinks that waking a patient and exposing him or her to very bright light at a critical moment in the early morning hours might jolt the internal clock and relieve the depression.

In Dr. Kripke's study, 12 depressed patients agreed to be awakened at odd hours of the night for one hour at a time on three consecutive nights. On one of the nights, the researchers woke them between one and two hours before their usual time of arising and exposed them to a very bright white fluorescent light. On a second night, the procedure was the same, but this time the patients were exposed to a dim red light. On the third night, they were awakened two to three hours *after retiring* and were exposed to a dim red light. Based on follow-up testing, the bright fluorescent light, used in the early morning, "significantly lowered their despression scores" temporarily (*Psychopharmacology Bulletin,* vol. 19, no. 3, 1983).

Whether these findings can be translated into information that health-minded people can use on their own remains to be seen. "It's all very interesting, it's promising and I'm excited by it from a scientific point of view," Dr. Kripke says. "But we are in the early stages of this and we aren't sure what the practical applications may be."

In the foregoing experiments, light was used to rouse and activate depressed persons. In other cases, certain parts of the light spectrum have been used to calm down hyperactive children. John Ott has maintained for several years that the cool-white fluorescent lights customarily used in elementary school classrooms contribute to hyperactivity and restlessness among the children. Part of the problem, he thought, was the fact that the tubes emit x-rays and harmful radio frequencies but do not emit the ultraviolet wavelengths that are found in sunlight. (Ott adds that fixtures have since been developed that remedy this problem.)

The wisdom of increasing our exposure to ultraviolet light has been hotly debated. According to Wendon Henton, Ph.D., of the National Center for Devices and Radiological Health, there have been claims that ultraviolet light can increase calcium absorption in the elderly and relieve headaches and fatigue.

Others have warned that the same band of light can cause cataracts and premature aging of the skin.

To researchers in the field, all of this means that we should pay much closer attention to the ways we use light. "There will have to be a reevaluation of the way we light our homes and offices and factories," said one government researcher. And there's a sense that we should waste no more time taking light for granted.

As Dr. Wurtman has pointed out, "Light is potentially too useful an agency of human health not to be more effectively examined and exploited."

Oral Hygiene Newsfront

Dental News Update

She was 40 years old, and there wasn't a cavity in her mouth because she brushed her teeth so well. Too well.

The problem was that over the years she'd scrubbed away at her teeth with such a vengeance that she'd finally brushed right through their hard surface. Her toothbrush had actually filed deep triangular grooves in her teeth right at the gum line.

Three teeth had become abscessed, their soft inner pulp exposed, and would need both root canal work and crowns. Many others would have to be filled with bonding materials if they were to be saved. It was going to cost a lot of money, which was something this woman didn't have. It meant she could lose all her teeth.

"This woman was a compulsive tooth brusher," says Laurence Fields, D.D.S., a Gaithersburg, Maryland, dentist interested in preventive dentistry. "While it's common to see tooth abrasion in patients because of faulty technique, it usually takes years to develop and is seldom permitted to become this severe."

People with dental abrasion can't be accused of neglecting their teeth. They often brush twice or more a day. Their brushing technique, however, leaves much to be desired. Doctors discovered why one man's teeth were almost hanging by threads when they asked him to show them how he brushed. The man used so much force he bent the handle of his toothbrush!

"I call it the 'dental chainsaw massacre,'" says Michael Lerner, D.M.D., a Lexington, Kentucky, dentist who sees signs of abrasion in about one-third of his new patients. "People literally injure tissues. It's as if you wanted to clean your fingers thoroughly and you decided to use sandpaper to do it. You could get the dirt off but you would also lose some skin.

"Some people have so equated cleanliness with health that they feel they have to brush their teeth after every meal or snack. But it takes 24 hours for bacteria to form acid-producing, cavity-causing plaque, so they may be going through a process that is unnecessary, although from a hygiene standpoint it might seem desirable. They are paying the price for cleanliness because they are sawing into their teeth."

The scene is set with a too-firm toothbrush and a horizontal, across-the-teeth brushing motion. "People get into the habit of brushing back and forth because it's easiest to do," Dr. Lerner says. "Maybe they've never learned the best way to brush their teeth—or the long-term consequences of bad brushing."

First, the brush begins to wear away the skin of the gums faster than it can grow back. When the gum has receded slightly, the root of the tooth is exposed. The root is not protected by enamel. It is covered with a thin protective substance called cementum, which quickly wears away. Beneath it is the dentin, a substance that makes up the bulk of the tooth and is similar to enamel but not as hard. Once the dentin comes in contact with your toothbrush and paste, your tooth can wear away 25 times more quickly.

For many people, the first sign of trouble is teeth that have become achingly sensitive to sweets, cold drinks and acidy foods like soft drinks or orange juice.

While there aren't any actual nerve endings in the dentin, there are tiny capillary-like tubules that carry fluids through the dentin to the outside and carry sensations inside to the tooth's nerve center. The tubules are sensitive to chemical changes on the surface of the tooth caused by some foods, and the response is felt as pain. The tooth's sensitivity to cold, though, occurs when it loses its insulation—when the enamel or dentin becomes too thin to adequately protect the pulp from temperature changes.

But the tooth does have the ability to become less sensitive, given half a chance. When the dentin is exposed, the pulp responds by laying down new dentin from within, building up "insulation" from the inside of the tooth and making its own chamber smaller. "The way I explain this process," Dr. Lerner says, "is, if someone cut a big hole in the roof of your home, you could at least add plaster to your ceiling. It would make the room a little smaller, but at least it would try to protect you from outside irritation."

The tubules will also seal themselves off at the tooth surface, but only if your brushing technique changes. "People who continue to brush too hard horizontally are slicing through the tubules every day. The tubules remain open and sensitive," Dr. Lerner says.

Dental abrasion will make you lose your teeth only in extreme cases, like the woman who brushed right down to the pulp. But it can contribute to gumline cavities and gum disease by making it easier for bacteria to accumulate.

Abraded areas make ideal "food traps," says Thomas McGuire, D.D.S., a California dentist and the author of *The Tooth Trip* (Random House). "Food is permitted to get in between the gums and teeth. It makes it more difficult to keep the mouth clean because the food can go into places it normally didn't. It means usually people have to start changing their brushing habits because what they used to do isn't going to be as effective any more."

Indeed, a change in brushing habits is all a case of dental abrasion often requires. While neither the enamel nor the gums will grow back, the dentin will desensitize slightly on its own. Calcium and other minerals found in saliva will help coat the tooth surface.

Fluoride applied to the dentin will also coat and help make it less sensitive. Dr. Lerner will sometimes coat teeth with a fluoride-containing desensitizing solution, which helps to remineralize the surface. He also gives patients fluoride gel to apply at home with a cotton swab. And both he and Dr. McGuire make sure their patients start brushing right.

One of the methods they teach is the widely recommended Bass Technique, a way of brushing that cleans your teeth thoroughly, especially around the gum line, with no danger of abrasion.

With this technique, patients use a small-headed toothbrush with soft, rounded-end or "polished" nylon bristles arranged in a straight line. They place the bristles at a 45-degree angle at the point where the teeth meet the gums, gently pushing the top row of bristles into the space between the tooth and gums. Then they wiggle or vibrate the bristles back and forth slightly, with firm pressure but very little horizontal motion of the toothbrush.

"I don't try to get every patient following these techniques perfectly," Dr. McGuire says. "What I try to do is to come up with something that works for them—something that keeps their teeth clean without doing them any harm. Brushing techniques have to be adapted to each person's mouth. And brushing alone isn't going to do it. You have to use dental floss, and, in some cases, a water pick."

"I try to get people to think of brushing their teeth as though they were scrubbing the wall right near a shag carpet," Dr. Lerner says. "They should try to scrub the wall but not the carpet itself. They want to picture the bristles of the brush as going right down to the edge of the floor, with the carpet just kind of gently pushed out of the way. The brushing pressure is directed toward the tooth, not the sensitive gum tissues."

Since it takes about 24 hours for new bacteria to form into plaque, Dr. Lerner has his patients brush thoroughly only once a day, using water. That way, he says, "You can feel with your tongue when your teeth are clean. They're not 'fuzzy' anymore. They're slick and smooth."

After meals, Dr. Lerner lets his patients brush only their chewing surfaces with a dab of toothpaste if they feel the need to do so.

All toothpastes are somewhat abrasive. That's what gives them their cleaning power. Abrasives scour off plaque, but they can also remove enamel, especially when you brush incorrectly. Toothpastes advertised as "stain-removing" or "smoker's toothpaste" are either excessively abrasive or acidic. So are baking soda and salt. "I know some people like to use baking soda, but I tell them to use it only occasionally, for instance, if they haven't had a chance to brush their teeth for more than 24 hours," Dr. McGuire says. "After all, people use it to scrub pots and pans."

Toothbrushes and toothpaste aren't the only things that can eat through enamel. Used in excess, acid foods like lemons, oranges, grapefruits, soda, vinegar—even the apples we thought were so good for our teeth, and their juice—can actually leach calcium out of the tightly packed crystal rods that form teeth enamel and, more important, erode the entire tooth structure. This can make it easier for plaque to form. Then the teeth feel gritty or rough, and their appearance changes from lustrous ivory to dull gray or yellow. Dentists call this process "erosion." They call any kind of mechanical wearing away, as in toothbrushing, "abrasion."

"Too much acid in the mouth dissolves the structure holding the crystals in place," Dr. Lerner says. "It's like pulling selected bricks out of a wall. You can pull some bricks out, and the wall will still stand. But if you keep pulling bricks out, eventually portions of the wall are going to break away."

There are some unusual causes of dental erosion. Some people have naturally acid saliva that eats their teeth away. Photoengravers and glass etchers often wear mouthguards because the acids and gritty materials they use in their work get into the air and on their front teeth.

Most cases of dental erosion, though, take place over several years and are caused by unusual eating habits. Sucking on lemons or drinking lemon juice every day is often to blame.

"Many of the cases you hear about are from Great Britain or Australia, where sipping warm lemon juice is seen as a great palliative for the common cold," says James L. Fuller, D.D.S., associate professor of operative dentistry at the University of Iowa.

But apparently it can happen much faster in some cases, as Dr. Fuller discovered when he treated a young woman who said her dental erosion had occurred overnight.

The enamel on the woman's front teeth and incisors was visibly pitted. "It looked like someone had shot them with very tiny buckshot," Dr. Fuller said.

The woman was positive her teeth had become scarred six years earlier during an all-night tequila-drinking bout. Following custom, the woman had "chased" her drinks by sucking on fresh lemon or lime halves. The next day, she said, she noticed the surface of her upper front teeth felt rough to her tongue.

"I was very surprised to find that such enamel damage could occur in so short a time," Dr. Fuller admits. "But if you know that citric acid was the first acid etch used to roughen up tooth enamel before plastic bonding material is applied, you realize the effect it can have on teeth."

The woman's teeth hadn't deteriorated further—but they had remained pitted. Dr. Fuller applied a bonding resin to protect the teeth and improve their appearance.

Taking your daily ration of vitamin C in a chewable tablet form can also cause enamel erosion, according to John Giunta, D.M.D., professor of oral pathology at Tufts University.

Dr. Giunta found severely eroded enamel on the teeth of a woman who had eaten three 500-milligram tablets of chewable vitamin C each day for three years. "Her teeth were actually getting shorter," Dr. Giunta says. "Up to one millimeter of enamel had been worn away in some areas, and several fillings were left standing higher than the tooth surface."

He found the pH of the tablets to be 1.92, about the same as stomach acid. A tooth placed in water containing a dissolved tablet became so soft its surface could be scratched away with a fingernail. "What you've got is a tablet of pure acid," Dr. Giunta says. "It just happens to be in a powder form, compacted. Of course, there's no problem if you swallow the tablets."

Chewing on aspirin tablets can cause the same sort of erosion, Dr. Giunta says. So can careless use of hydrochloric acid tablets or drops used to replace stomach acid.

It really doesn't matter what you are putting in your mouth, Dr. Giunta says. "If it has a pH of 5.5 or less, it can erode your teeth." Lemons have a pH of 2.1; pure lemon juice, 2.4; cola drinks, which contain carboxylic acid, 2.5; orange juice, lemonade and grapefruits, 2.7; grapefruit and lime juice, 2.9; vinegar, 3.1; and apple juice, 3.3.

"And you can't consider pH alone," Dr. Giunta says. "How much of these foods you eat is also important. If you drink 6 ounces of soda a day, you probably won't get any erosion. If you drink more than 12 ounces, there is the potential for erosion. Someone who drinks 24 ounces a day has a much greater likelihood of having this happen to his teeth."

What can you do to minimize the effects? Drink through a straw, for one thing, Dr. Giunta says. Simply chewing your citrus fruits instead of sucking on them may also help, says Dr. Fuller.

Dr. McGuire suggests rinsing your mouth well with plain water after eating acid foods. Baking soda is alkaline, with a pH of 8 to 9. Rinsing with it may help neutralize your mouth.

You may also want to wait to brush, since teeth are more prone to abrasion immediately after exposure to acid foods. It takes 20 minutes to an hour for the mouth to neutralize acid and minerals in the saliva to recoat the tooth.

And when you do brush, do it right. A thorough but gentle cleaning will add more miles to your smile than thoughtless hacking away.

What You Should Know about Root Canal Surgery

Suddenly you know you can't wait any longer. Your tooth is in labor and the whole side of your face is throbbing in response. The dentist confirms your worst fears—the nerve has died and become infected. It's root canal therapy or lose the tooth.

It's not as if you've never heard of this procedure before. It's that you've heard too much, and none of it good. Now it's time to learn for yourself—and not from somebody else's bad experience—just what to expect.

Ease up. The news is good. It's no longer a painful procedure and the success rate is high—about 94 percent.

But you need to know much more than that to ease your mind. That's where we come in. Our list of questions and answers covers all aspects of the procedure, including potential complications (yes, there are a few rare ones).

To help us we went to the experts, the dentists who specialize in root canal therapy, called endodontists. Donald

Arens, D.D.S., is an associate professor at the Indiana University School of Dentistry in Indianapolis and former president of the American Association of Endodontists. Michael Heuer, D.D.S., is a professor at Northwestern University School of Dentistry in Chicago and vice president of the American Association of Endodontists. And Irwin Smigel, D.D.S., a general dentist, is author of *Dental Health, Dental Beauty* (M. Evans, 1979) and a postgraduate lecturer at the New York University College of Dentistry.

What exactly is root canal therapy?

It's the complete removal of a tooth's nerve. That means the part that not only fills the hollow center of every tooth (crown), but also the parts that continue as canals down into the root (or roots) below the gum. The nerve is removed when it has died and becomes infected.

What causes the nerve to die?

Most often it's from a neglected cavity. Once decay has penetrated the dentin (the layer under the enamel) it can move on to the pulp (the center of the tooth, which contains the nerves and blood vessels). Now the nerve is exposed to germs and infection can set in causing an inflammation and swelling inside the canal. Since the root canal is rigid, this swelling strangles the pulp, cuts off its blood supply and kills it.

A trauma to the tooth, such as a severe blow or even excessive heat from a drill, can also cause irreversible nerve damage. If blood flow (and the oxygen it carries) to the nerve is interrupted, the nerve begins to die. Dr. Smigel compares it to stroke victims whose oxygen to the brain is temporarily cut off. Brain cells die, often leaving permanent damage, just like with the nerve of a tooth.

Why does the tooth hurt if the nerve is dead?

A nerve that has died almost always becomes abscessed. Eventually the gases that build up inside the canal burst through the bottom of the root, deep in the gum, spreading infection and pus to surrounding areas. While the dead nerve *inside* the canal is no longer causing pain, the nerves in the jawbone and in the *outer* covering of the root (cementum) are still alive — and surely let you know it.

Can I have a dead nerve without pain?

Yes. While the nerve is dying, there is usually a great deal of pain. But it disappears completely after the nerve has died. It's actually possible to go years without further trouble—but it's unlikely. That's because bacteria love to munch on the dead pulp and sooner or later (usually sooner) it will abscess.

How can a dentist be sure that my problem is caused by a dying or dead nerve?

The dentist will conduct a few very simple tests on the tooth in question as well as the teeth surrounding the "bad" one. First he will see how your teeth respond to heat, then cold, and finally to an electrical pulp tester that sends a low current through the tooth.

In a normal, healthy tooth, you should be able to feel the heat, cold and electrical current as clearly uncomfortable— meaning the nerve is alive and well. Of course the dentist stops as soon as you signal that you've felt it. Then the discomfort should stop immediately, too.

All normal teeth should respond similarly, so that a tooth that dosen't becomes suspect. For example, a tooth whose nerve is in the process of dying shows a lower level of current. Ice causes pain that persists after it's removed and then gradually goes away. Heat, on the other hand, causes a *severe* toothache that can actually be relieved by something cold.

If the nerve is completely dead, you will not feel anything at all when the tooth is tested.

"These tests are very valuable," Dr. Heuer explains, "but they are not foolproof. I'd say they're about 75 to 80 percent accurate, so it's important for your dentist to use other diagnostic tools as well. Is there a deep filling? Has there been a trauma to the tooth? What does the x-ray show? Has there been pain on previous occasions? Then he will be better able to make a correct diagnosis."

How is root canal therapy done?

Very carefully. The dentist uses a mechanical drill only to clean out the nerve in the crown of the tooth, but then uses hand instruments for the rest of the procedure. These instruments, called reamers and broaches, range in size from tiny to tinier, depending on the size of the canal they must be inserted into. By twisting and thrusting these instruments into the canal, the dentist is able to remove all of its contents. Meanwhile, the canals are continuously flushed to remove debris. After that canals are smoothed and shaped with special files to prepare them for the filling material.

The preferred filling, Dr. Smigel told us, is gutta-percha, a natural rubberlike substance derived from the sap of a tropical tree. It shapes itself to fit the inside of the canal and seals off the tip of the root completely. It can also be easily removed if the root canal has to be reworked for some reason.

The other material that is sometimes used is silver point filling. But this is "difficult, if not impossible," to remove once it's in place, and it doesn't create as good a seal, explains Dr. Smigel.

How does the dentist know if he has filled all the canals in a tooth?

It's tricky, all right. Because even though certain teeth have a particular number of roots (from one to three, depending on the tooth) a root may actually have more than one canal. And every one must be cleaned thoroughly to the bottom and then filled. Since the dentist is working in the dark (so to speak), he must rely on precision instruments and x-rays to see if he's reached the bottom.

How many visits to the dentist does it take to complete the root canal therapy?

Usually three. The roots are completely cleaned out and sterilized on the first visit. A temporary filling is put in but sometimes an opening is left for drainage if the infection is severe.

The second appointment seems a lot like the first, but actually the dentist is cleaning the canals even more thoroughly and is shaping them in preparation for the filling.

At the third and final visit, the dentist puts in the gutta-percha filling.

Why do the root canals have to be filled?

"It's the old story of 'nature abhors a vacuum,'" Dr. Smigel points out. "If the dentist doesn't fill the canals after the nerve has been removed, the body will fill them itself—with bacteria."

It's also part of what Dr. Arens calls "the triad of success. Get to the bottom of the root, clean it out completely and make it solid to keep out germs."

Can root canal therapy be done successfully on any tooth?

No. Some teeth have roots that are so crooked or so narrow that inserting the reamers to the bottom is virtually impossible. And cleaning out only the part of the root that can be reached will never do. Any nerve material left inside becomes the next main course for bacteria.

Also, the roots of very old teeth sometimes become calcified and so hardened that even a hammer and chisel won't budge them.

Even when root canal therapy can be completed (which is most of the time), there is still a slight chance that it won't correct the problem.

What can be done next, short of losing the tooth?

When infection persists despite completion of the root canal (pain will tell you something is wrong), your dentist may recommend a procedure called an apicoectomy, which is done by an endodontist or oral surgeon. The still-infected roots are approached by cutting through the gum and bone between the root and cheek. The surgeon exposes the root, cleans out the infection and sometimes cuts off the tips of the infected roots to make sure the source of the infection is gone — permanently. The ends of the roots are then sealed off with a filling material.

For people whose roots are too crooked, too narrow or have become calcified, there is yet another option, Dr. Arens explains. "We can extract the problem tooth, clean and seal the roots and then replant it in the mouth—all within 30 minutes. A temporary splint is required to hold it in place," says Dr. Arens. "The success rate is 80 percent, not quite as high as conventional root canal therapy, but it's better than losing the tooth."

How much does root canal therapy cost?

It varies depending on the tooth involved. After all, much more work is required in a tooth with three roots than in a tooth with just one. The cost can also vary depending on what part of the country you live in. Generally you can figure on about $175 for the simplest case to about $500 for a more complex problem. To be sure, ask your own dentist.

It's likely however, that pulling the tooth and replacing it with a false tooth or bridge would be far more expensive.

Our Changing Medical System

"7-11 Medicine": A Controversial New Approach to Convenience

It's Sunday evening and that respiratory infection you've been battling all week has just called up reinforcements. It's germ warfare, and your body's losing.

Think fast: Should you call your doctor? You can't. His hours are 9 to 5, weekdays only. Should you drive to the hospital emergency room? No. It's 20 miles away and three times as expensive as your family physician. Besides, the last time you were there you had to wait four hours while the medical team sewed up crash victims and screened drug addicts.

You've got it: You'll zip down to the shopping mall and pop into the walk-in medical center. You'll be diagnosed, treated and back home in 30 minutes flat.

Walk-in medical center? It sounds like something that's been around ever since physicians stopped making house calls, but walk-in centers offering all-around doctoring are about as newfangled as you can get in American health care.

To the dismay of many private practitioners and the delight

of thousands of patients, walk-in medical centers (often called freestanding emergency centers) have evolved into a whole new breed of medical practice—a cross between the family physician and the hospital emergency room. Like your local M.D., the centers treat pains, fevers, cuts and breaks (everything but life-threatening emergencies). And like an emergency room, they have extended hours (most are open 12 to 14 hours per day) and no appointments.

And don't look now, but such a novelty may have just cropped up in your neighborhood. There are over 1,100 of them coast to coast, and they're opening up at the rate of at least one a day. Last year probably as many as 25 million people bypassed family doctors and hospital emergency rooms to get medical help in these centers, and this year the numbers are likely to be larger.

The force behind the trend is easy enough to identify, say the advocates of walk-in medicine: The centers exist because people need and want them.

"People don't use health care the way they used to," says James R. Roberts, executive director of the National Association of Freestanding Emergency Centers. "The consumer now demands medical treatment that's more accessible and more affordable, and these centers help meet those requirements."

"There's a clear need for convenient, consumer-oriented quality care," says Joseph G. Maloney, M.D., vice president of a chain of walk-in centers in the Boston area. "In no other industry is the relationship between the consumer and the provider as unbalanced as in health care. You wait for a week for an appointment, and then the average waiting time in a doctor's office is one hour. If the doctor's office is closed, you go to the emergency room and wait until the life-and-death emergency cases are taken care of. Any dry cleaner that operated this way would be put out of business."

Critics of the centers, on the other hand, see them as an awkward step in precisely the wrong direction. They believe that walk-in clinics probably provide questionable health care ("Docs-in-a-Box" and "7-Eleven Medicine" are favorite epithets), and that they break up the "continuity of care" offered by family doctors.

True or false? It may be too early to tell. But we think we uncovered some clues when we took a firsthand look at Dr. Maloney's half dozen walk-ins that dot the Boston suburbs.

Called Health Stop, they have all the consumer conveniences that their slick moniker implies. Scrubbed and spacious facilities (with examination rooms, waiting areas, conference rooms, x-ray rooms, even children's play areas) announce themselves where the people are—suburban thoroughfares and shopping centers. At each clinic, two full-time doctors and about ten full- or part-time nurses and medical assistants treat patients without appointments seven days a week, 8 A.M. to 9 P.M. And they do so with impressive efficiency: Patients are greeted within 30 seconds after they walk through the door and are seen by a doctor within 15 minutes.

"Patients seem to like what we're doing here," says C. Matthew Masserman, M.D., medical director at one of the centers. "So far, feedback from patients has been almost all positive."

Other Health Stop physicians report much the same. And considering the wide spectrum of care the doctors offer, such blessings from their patients may be some kind of record.

"We're a doctor's office with extended capabilities," Dr. Maloney says. "People can come to us because they have a sore throat or fracture or want a physical exam, and we can diagnose swiftly because we have laboratory and x-ray equipment on the premises. We practice general medicine with a consumerist twist."

What they don't do, however, is pretend to be an emergency room capable of handling crises that threaten life and limb. And neither do most other walk-in medical centers. Like other walk-ins, Health Stop clinics don't accept ambulances. And the word "emergency" (used warily in half the other 1,100 walk-ins) has become a no-no among Health Stop's marketing and medical pesonnel.

It's just as well. The word, and the idea it conveys, has been the focus of criticism of walk-in centers everywhere. Some physicians charge that, whether or not "emergency" is on a walk-in's shingle, it's too easy for a critically ill patient to run to a walk-in medical center when he should be hurrying to a hospital emergency room. The detour, they say, could be fatal.

Doctors at walk-ins counter that they go out of their way to help people make the distinction between the two kinds of care. Besides, they say, if somebody with a life-threatening medical emergency does show up at the door, they're trained and equipped to stabilize him and transport him to the hospital.

"Like most other walk-in centers," says Dr. Maloney, "each Health Stop is equipped with oxygen gear, defibrillator, crash cart [mobile emergency medicine chest], monitors and more. We're ready for serious medical problems should they arise. And once in a while they do arise, just as they do in a doctor's office. The difference is we're ready, and some doctors' offices aren't."

How walk-in medical centers handle more routine health problems, though, may be a better test of the quality of their care. At Health Stop, at least, there are signs that the analogies to fast food stores are wide of the mark.

"We've taken steps to ensure that the consumer gets his money's worth," Dr. Maloney says. "We've staffed the centers with the most qualified physicians we could find. We make sure that all x-rays and cardiograms are double-checked by radiologists and cardiologists. Four of our centers are affiliated with hospitals to augment our medical services. And every month we submit staff doctors to a rigorous review by a committee of their peers. The committee ensures that doctors aren't overtesting or overmedicating, that they're treating patients correctly and consistently."

Antique Medicine
Is Alive and Dangerous

From medicine man to apothecary to brain surgeon, the aim has always been true: to heal the body of disease and relieve pain. But the ways of healing change from generation to generation, as scientists continually introduce new treatments and discard old, disproven ones. So what once was hailed as the latest in modern medicine simply may no longer work . . . and perhaps never did.

Take tonsillectomies. Doctors used to eliminate your chronic throat problems by eliminating your tonsils. They discovered, however, that it was not only unnecessary but could also weaken your body's defenses. Since then, routine tonsillectomies have gone the way of house calls and little black bags. According to the National Center for Health Statistics, over 1.2 million tonsillectomies were performed in 1965, but only 457,000 were done in 1981.

Still, there are numerous "routine" practices that are alive and kicking in hospitals and doctor's offices—practices that have little or no scientific basis and that probably should be retired.

Shaving before Surgery

Hospital patients, in preparation for surgery, are usually shaved in the area that will be operated on. Since doctors consider hair a source of contamination, this procedure is meant to lower the chances of infection after the operation, as well as to clear the skin for surgical work. But is clean-cut necessarily cleaner? The evidence says no, according to an editorial in *Lancet* (June 11, 1983).

In one study, a researcher examined a group that was scheduled for abdominal surgery. The patients were divided into three groups: shaved, treated with hair-removal cream and unshaved. After the operations, wound infections appeared in 12.4 percent of shaved patients, 7.9 percent of those treated with the cream and only 7.8 percent of those who weren't shaved.

Most surgeons have their patients shaved as much as 24 hours before an operation. But studies show that the longer the interval between shaving and surgery, the more bacteria there will be on the skin. If more than 24 hours pass between shaving and surgery, the post-surgical infection rate can rise as high as 20 percent. A delay makes no difference when hair-removal cream is used.

Cola for Sick Children

Pediatricians often recommend cola for children with mild dehydration caused by stomach or intestinal disorder. The soda is prescribed to replenish water and replace potassium, which helps maintain the balance of fluids in the body. But a closer look by a Swiss researcher shows that two prominent colas and a noncola soft drink contain only tiny amounts, less than 2 milligrams per ounce, of potassium. And the small amounts found in these soft drinks most likely come from the water that's used as an ingredient (*Lancet*, February 26, 1983). Fruit juices, however, are high in potassium. Frozen apple juice mixes to about 38 milligrams of potassium per ounce, and frozen orange juice has about 59 milligrams per ounce.

So when it comes to sick children, it seems Coke isn't it, after all.

Routine Chest X-rays

Remember that small dose of radiation "just to check if you're okay" that you got as part of your company's health examination? It was required for the job, so you went along with it.

Scenes like that may be changing, however, as more studies show that too few cases of chest and lung disease are detected in diagnostic x-rays to justify the cost and added radiation exposure for people without symptoms. The American College of Radiology (ACR) recently recommended that chest x-rays no longer be included in routine prenatal examinations, hospital admissions, tuberculosis screenings and preemployment examinations.

Many companies still require chest x-rays for new employees as a part of periodic health exams, but more firms are eliminating them from routine checkups. The ACR also says that employees who are exposed at work to dangerous substances, such as asbestos, and are thus at higher risk of contracting disease, should still be x-rayed periodically. However, these x-rays should be scheduled according to the length of time between initial exposure to a dangerous substance and the earliest possible onset of disease—for asbestosis, this is normally no less than ten years. Smokers exposed to asbestos may need x-rays sooner and more frequently, since smoking compounds the effects.

Employees whose companies pay for their health exams should be extra-careful about diagnostic x-rays. Many firms hire clinics to administer these checkups. In order to charge high fees, the clinics sometimes include as many tests as they can. This may mean exposure to radiation that can do more harm than good.

Most chest x-rays test for tuberculosis or lung cancer, although they can detect other problems, such as change in heart size, rib abnormalities and benign lung lesions. But by the time lung cancer has advanced enough to show up on an x-ray, it's usually too late to cure it. For tuberculosis, an x-ray should be taken only if a preliminary skin test is positive.

Some physicians include an upper gastrointestinal (GI) series in routine exams. This is an expensive test for stomach cancer, ulcers and other abdominal disorders, in which the patient swallows barium before taking an x-ray. Since the radiation dose is relatively high, the upper GI series is useful only for people who already have symptoms.

Radical Mastectomies

A decade ago, if you were unfortunate enough to have a malignant breast tumor, you were practically certain to be a candidate for a radical mastectomy. It was a dear price to pay, but the operation was trusted as the best bet for survival.

But no more. Statistics show that the radical mastectomy which involves removal of the breast, chest muscle and underarm lymph nodes, has not brought much higher survival rates than a less extreme method called a modified radical mastectomy.

A federal panel of experts at the National Institutes of Health a few years ago recommended the *modified* radical mastectomy as the current standard of treatment for women with early signs of breast cancer, rather than the traditional radical mastectomy. This less-disfiguring operation involves removal of the breast and lymph nodes, but leaves the under-lying chest muscles intact.

Fortunately, this new standard seems to have been quickly adopted. About 200,000 medical records from approximately 400 hospitals across the country are surveyed annually by the National Center for Health Statistics. The results show that, of all mastectomies performed from 1972 to 1974, 48.5 percent were radical; from 1975 to 1977, the number decreased to 31 percent; and from 1978 to 1980, only 14.2 percent of all mastectomies were radical.

Carol Case, director of the Breast Cancer Education Program at the National Cancer Institute, says that even less severe surgical procedures are currently being tested. "One of the newest procedures is the lumpectomy, where only the tumor is removed. If it proves malignant, partial or complete removal of the underarm lymph nodes may follow, and the breast may then be treated with radiation therapy," she says. This allows a woman to keep the affected breast and spares her some of the trauma of breast cancer.

Ms. Case adds that while studies are not yet complete, the preliminary results look very promising.

In addition, a major study at the National Cancer Institute in Milan, Italy, reported that women with small breast tumors (less than two centimeters) who had only a fourth of the breast removed and then received radiation treatment survived as long as women who underwent radical mastectomies (*New England Journal of Medicine,* July 2, 1982). This study and others like it are proving that radical mastectomies are needlessly drastic and should be performed only on the occasional patient whose cancer has spread to the chest muscles.

Annual Physicals

Once thought of as a milestone in preventive health care, the expensive yearly checkup is losing out to wiser, more cost-effective health programs geared to more specific needs. Instead of automatically ordering a battery of laboratory tests and x-rays, more and more doctors are opting for periodic screening tests based on age, sex, lifestyle and family history.

The idea of routine checkups was based on the assumption that early detection, diagnosis and treatment of chronic diseases could reduce complications later. But discovering serious illnesses in routine exams is rare, and most young, low-risk patients walk out of their doctor's office with a clean bill of health. For the small percentage of cancer and diabetes diagnosed in presymptomatic stages, there's no proof that early treatment has decreased mortality.

The Canadian Task Force on the Periodic Health Examination did a three-year study on the value of annual exams, and reported that the "routine general annual checkup is nonspecific and casts a searching net too broadly, particularly in the adult, is inefficient and, at times, is potentially harmful" (*World Health Forum,* vol. 2, no. 1, 1981).

The committee recommended that the annual physical be replaced by a selective periodic health examination gauged to a person's age and sex. For example, a woman in her childbearing years should have a Pap smear annually and a breast exam periodically to supplement home checks for lumps. Women over 50 years old should routinely have a mammogram to check for breast cancer. All adults over 45 years old should be screened regularly for colon cancer, and those over 35 should check for glaucoma about every three years.

Most of these tests can be done when a patient visits his doctor for illness-related treatment.

Enemas during Labor

It has been established practice in many hospitals to give an enema to expectant mothers just before birth. The contractions during labor often cause women to lose control of their bowels. Emptying the bowels supposedly lowers the chance of fecal contamination and infection during birth. Also some obstetricians and midwives believe that without an enema, labor would be prolonged and more difficult.

But a study of 274 women showed that none of these assumptions was true. Enema or no enema, 84 percent of the expectant mothers had no problems with contamination in the first stage of labor. In the second stage of labor, 65 percent of patients who had enemas and 61 percent of those who didn't had clean deliveries (*British Medical Journal,* April 18, 1981).

A New Code
of Practice for Doctors

The People's Medical Society, a new
nonprofit group, is asking physicians to
show their clients a little more respect.

Imagine this: You walk into you doctor's office and check
in with the receptionist. You're immediately ushered into an
examining room. A couple of minutes later, the doctor comes
in. He sits down and asks you about your symptoms, listening
intently. After an examination, he sits down again and discusses
the diagnosis with you. He describes the tests that might help
confirm it, what each will tell you, what they're like and what
they'll cost. He also explains your treatment alternatives, the
cost of each, the side effects, if any, and the chances of
success. He clearly answers all of your questions, making sure
you fully understand the implications of each option. Then he
asks *you* a question: "What do you want to do?"

Sounds like a dream, right? Well, you don't have to imagine
it, because across the country, doctors are actually signing
their names to a code that says they will conduct their practice
in a manner based on the principles of open communication
and respect for each patient.

Developed by the People's Medical Society (PMS), a
55,000-member consumer organization founded by Robert
Rodale, the Code of Practice is a ten-point statement, to be
endorsed by doctors, of just what health-care consumers expect
and demand from medical practitioners.

"We felt it was necessary to make a clear statement, up
front, to the medical profession about how we, the consumers
of health care, want the doctor-patient relationship to be,"
explains Charles Inlander, executive director of the People's
Medical Society, a non-profit, independent organization. "So
we looked at our mail, at that point approximately 20,000
letters, and it was very clear. Ten things stood out that consumers were angry about or didn't like. They concerned two general areas: office procedures and choices in diagnosis and

treatment. So when we drafted the Code, we decided to orga-
nize it that way."

The first half of the Code reflects consumers' dissatisfac-
tion with some of the nonmedical aspects of doctor-patient
interaction, such as having to wait too long or being shocked
by the bill. The second half stems from complaints that doctors
aren't giving their patients enough information about their
condition and their medical options.

"The key point is that the Code does not require doctors
to alter the way they do medicine," says Inlander. But it may
require them to alter the way they deal with patients.

"We're not suggesting that the doctor do an angioplasty
instead of a bypass," he explains. "What we are saying is 'tell
me what my options are and let me make the decisions. In
other words, give me information. It is incumbent upon you to
do that in order for me to make an informed choice.' The
bottom line of all this is that we believe the doctor-patient
relationship should be a partnership. The Code of Practice is
the standard by which we can measure whether a doctor
believes in a partnership approach to health care."

So how do you know if a doctor endorses the Code? "To
start out, we did a test in Palm Beach County, Florida," Inlander
explains. "We publicized the Code on television, radio and in
the newspapers. At the same time, we mailed copies of the
Code of Practice to all 1,200 medical practitioners in the
county, asking them to sign it. Forty-seven doctors did.

"On the one hand, that's pretty disappointing. But it's not
a failure on our part. We feel it's a failure of the medical
system. On the other hand, the citizens of Palm Beach County
are the only ones in the country who know 47 doctors who are
willing to stand out and say 'I believe in consumerism. I'm very
willing to follow these standards. There's nothing unreason-
able about this Code and I'm willing to put my name down
on it.' "

To spread the word in the rest of the country, PMS members are bringing the Code to their doctors personally and
asking them to sign. The PMS keeps a list of all the doctors
who've endorsed the Code, so members can easily obtain the

names of doctors in their area who subscribe to its principles. And they're finding that many doctors do.

"I do all of those things," says Irving Lang, M.D., an obstetrician from Fort Lauderdale, Florida, who endorses the Code. "It's just good medicine. In fact, the Code should say I *do*, not I will."

In fact, most doctors who've signed the Code say they've always followed its principles. "Patient education has been the focus of my whole practice for 25 years," says Walt Stoll, M.D., founder and medical director of the Holistic Health Center in Lexington, Kentucky. "The patient is the most important member of the health-care team. The physician is just a consultant in how you run your life. People *should* be more involved in their treatment." And if the number of PMS members is any indication, that's just what many people are looking for.

"I want to know as much about what's happening to me as I can," says Alma Rose, a PMS member from Palm Beach Gardens, Florida. "If I have heart disease or cancer, it's not the doctor's problem, it's mine. I'd at least like to have a hand in the decisions, and an educated decision is better than a wild stab. The less you know about what's happening to you, the more you become a sacrificial offering. It's incredible, yet many people voluntarily climb up on a table and are cut open without first knowing all of the other options."

According to the Code, it's not just knowing what your choices are, it's knowing exactly what each entails.

"I've always been especially careful about informing the patient," says Joel F. Spatt, D.P.M., a subscriber to the Code from Hoffman Estates, Illinois. "I let them know exactly what to expect. If they're considering a surgical procedure, I'll actually *draw* it for them, because it can be difficult to comprehend if you only tell them verbally.

"It's been my experience that if you're confused, you won't do well. The psychological part is very important in rehabilitation," he explains. "Besides, I owe it to patients. They're human beings. Why aren't they entitled to know what I'm going to do to their bodies? I feel it's their innate right."

Dr. Stoll concurs. "It's important for the patient to know

exactly what to expect. For instance, if a patient has pneumonia, I'll actually give them written information that tells them which symptoms are usual and which aren't. It eases their minds and makes them calmer. That way they also know when something is wrong and they should call me.

"When I first started practicing, I was getting a tremendous number of phone calls at night," Dr. Stoll told us. "Then I began an effort to educate the patients, and things changed drastically. Within six months the number of calls dropped from 50 a week to 2 or 3 a week. It's not that I mind the calls. The point is that the patients are calmer and there are less unnecessary visits." For the patients, that means fewer unnecessary expenses.

And with the high cost of medical care these days, many people would be wise to know their financial options as well as their treatment options, a subject addressed by the first point of the Code.

"Many doctors have commented that it's sort of merchandising themselves," says PMS's Inlander. "Well, that's exactly what we want. How can we shop if we don't know what the fees are ahead of time? And I think we *should* shop for price." To many people, knowing whether the doctor is going to charge $25 or $50 for an office visit can be a deciding factor.

"Some people don't have insurance, so they really need to know," says Mrs. Rose. "I just like to have a good ballpark figure up front."

"The list doesn't have to be detailed down to the price of a tongue depressor," adds Michael Rooney, director of planning for PMS. "We just want doctors to give people a general idea."

"I always like patients to know the fees in advance," Dr. Spatt told us. "There's nothing worse than when a patient hadn't the faintest idea of what it was going to cost."

"I don't know why doctors would object to it," says Richard Tapert, D.O., of the Family Health Clinic in Detroit. "The list of fees is generally available anyway. You need it for when insurance companies are paying for some of the services."

Another important point of the Code that many doctors object to is bringing someone into the examining room with you. "I could be cynical and say that perhaps those doctors don't want witnesses, but more likely they think it takes away from the privacy of the doctor-patient relationship," says Inlander. "Really we're suggesting that you *do* have a witness in the room. The reason is that you're going in very vulnerable. You're sick. You're not feeling well. You're scared. You either forget to ask a lot of the questions you have or you don't hear what the doctor says. It's another set of ears and another mouth in the room with you, and we feel it's very important."

For two groups of doctors, such a policy is routine. Obstetricians are used to having husbands in the examining room for their wives' prenatal visits and all the way through delivery. They don't question it. Neither do pediatricians. Obviously, an infant or toddler must be accompanied.

"But adults are supposed to have it together all the time. Well, even adults can be incapacitated when they're sick," says Sandra Thomas, a PMS member from Delray Beach, Florida.

"The real question is, why doesn't that practitioner want to facilitate an exchange of information?" Rooney points out. "Why doesn't he want to make sure that the patient understands and hears everything he says?"

"I give patients a lot of information and lifestyle advice," Dr. Stoll told us. "So it's helpful to have another person there who's willing to help. We encourage it."

And there are other good reasons why a person might want company in the examining room. "I find that a lot of people like to bring someone with them for support," says Dr. Spatt. "And frankly if the patient is calmer, it works to my benefit. I never prevent anyone from coming in, even friends. Patients do better with moral support."

Dr. Lang agrees. "I get every Aunt Tillie and Uncle George in here at one time or another. It doesn't bother me at all. And if it reassures the patient, it's helpful."

It can also be helpful and reassuring to have a copy of your medical records. The Code provides for that, too. "I want to see the doctor's evaluation of my medical condition," says Miss Thomas. "And I want a file of my records in my home. I want to have them in case I decide to change doctors, get a second opinion or see a specialist."

"Sometimes it can help the doctor to make a diagnosis if

he has your old records for comparison," adds Mrs. Rose. "If I move, I've got them. If there's an emergency, I've got them. Besides, who knows what's on your records? If you don't check, you don't know."

"There's nothing in the Code you wouldn't expect in any other consumer situation," Miss Thomas points out. "People won't put up with that stuff in a restaurant, for instance. If a waitress is rude, you report her to the manager. But when it comes to health care, people are afraid and intimidated. They'll keep going back to a doctor even though he or she treats them poorly."

"Medicine is the last bastion of nonconsumerism," says Inlander. "The PMS is showing doctors that there's a viable group of consumers out there, growing at a rate of 1,000 new members a week, who are not going to tolerate this anymore.

"The Code of Practice lays it out the medical world: For the first time in the history of modern medicine, the consumer is stepping forward in an organized way and saying, 'It's going to be done the way we want. We're paying the bills and they're our bodies. No longer are you the one who's going to ordain how it's going to be. We'll tell *you* how it's going to be.' "

Prescription for Addiction
Street drugs aren't the only kind that can lead to addiction.

They had sweet little names like "Mrs. Winslow's Soothing Syrup," "Ayer's Cherry Pectoral" or "Godfrey's Cordial," and they were sold all over the country a century ago. Their manufacturers claimed they could work magic on everything from a bad cold to consumption—and there really *was* some sort of magic in those odd-looking little bottles. Trouble was, it was often black magic, because "the nostrums of the great American medicine show during the 1800s brought more narcotics like opium and morphine into American homes than all the modern-day hard-drug dealers combined," says Stephen J. Levy, Ph.D., author of *Managing the Drugs in Your Life*

(McGraw-Hill, 1983). Accounts from that period estimated that over 200,000 Americans had become addicted to the opium in those bottled cure-alls with the sweet little names.

All opiates were removed from over-the-counter remedies in 1914 (they're still available in some prescription medicines), so you and I have been protected from one of the most addictive drugs in the modern medicine chest. But today, the potential for becoming drug dependent is even greater than it was in the days of Godfrey's Cordial, because the number and variety of drugs has increased so dramatically.

The problem is complex and widespread. For one thing, we're a drug-dependent society encouraged to take some sort of medication for every ill. For another, it just isn't that easy to make certain drugs (like tranquilizers, painkillers and sleeping pills) completely nonaddictive, says Dr. Levy, who is executive director of the Institute on Alcoholism and Substance Abuse at City University of New York. "Quite a few analgesics [painkillers] were once promoted as nonaddicting narcotics but eventually turned out to lead to physical and psychological addiction," he told us. Among those drugs are Demerol, Dilaudid and Talwin.

You're probably in no danger of becoming a ragged, homeless addict if you find yourself regularly filling your prescription for these drugs. But there are many levels of drug dependence—what about taking a laxative every day or never leaving home without your antacids? To varying degrees, all can be unhealthy.

Generally, pharmacologists recognize three different kinds of drug dependence, Dr. Levy explains. You're *physically* addicted if you experience unpleasant "withdrawal" symptoms like nausea, headaches or the cold sweats when you don't take the drug; your dosage of the drug has also probably steadily increased over time. *Psychological* addiction, a bit more subtle, is the belief that you simply can't cope without the drug, and *functional* addiction is what happens when you use drugs like nasal decongestant sprays to relieve an annoying physical condition, then gradually grow dependent on the drugs to keep you free of the problem.

All these tidy distinctions really matter more to doctors

than to the rest of us—if you've grown drug dependent, you don't really care how or why. What's important is that it's all too easy, that it can happen to anyone, and that it can be damaging to your health.

"Caffeine is a perfect example of a drug that millions of people have become physically and psychologically addicted to," says Joe Graedon, pharmacologist and author of *The People's Pharmacy* (St. Martin's Press). "So many people believe they just can't function without that cup of coffee in the morning, and get the classic 'withdrawal headache' if they miss a day without it. People don't realize that many medicines also contain caffeine."

A relatively mild addiction, true. But if you think a drug has to be powerful—or illegal—to be addicting, you're wrong.

"There are far more people in this country who are having trouble with prescription drugs than with 'street drugs,' " Dr. Levy says. In fact, the federal Drug Abuse Warning Network reported that during 1980, 15 of the 20 "most abused" drugs were prescription drugs, many of them known to be habit forming. The prescription tranquilizer Valium was number one. Heroin was number two. Other top scorers: Methaqualone (sold under the brand names Quaalude, Parest and others), Dalmane, Placidyl and phenobarbital, all sleeping pills; Darvon, Talwin and Percodan, all mild analgesics; Tranxene and Librium, mild tranquilizers; and acetaminophen with codeine.

In her best-selling book *I'm Dancing As Fast As I Can* (Harper & Row), television producer Barbara Gordon told the terrifying story of her physical and mental collapse following "cold turkey" withdrawal from tranquilizers. "I had started taking Valium for a back problem, beginning with 4 milligrams a day," she writes. "Now I was up to 30 and couldn't get out of the house without taking them." Determined to be "free of pills," one day she simply quit. Her psychiatrist had told her repeatedly that the drug was not addicting, and when he learned of her plan to quit, failed to warn her that abuptly stopping the drug could produce physical side effects more wrenching than the withdrawal from heroin. When she tried it, her world simply fell apart.

Was it possible her doctor really didn't know the drug

could become addictive with long-term use? "Absolutely," contends Joan Levin, coauthor of *Stopping Valium* (Warner Books, 1983). The book, written partly in response to Ms. Gordon's story (with Sidney Wolf, M.D., and Eve Bargmann, M.D., of the Washington-based Public Citizen Health Research Group), contends that "many Americans who would never think of themselves as 'drug addicts' have gotten into trouble with prescription drugs simply by taking the advice of the good old family doctor."

The problem, Dr. Levy says, is that most of the drug education doctors get comes from drug companies, whose bias is obvious. "Practicing physicians, who are inadequately trained in pharmacology [drugs] in medical school, get most of their drug information from three sources, all provided by the drug companies," he says. "From advertisements in medical journals, from detail men [salesmen] who ply them with free samples and from the *Physician's Desk Reference* [or *PDR,* the so-called drug bible that lists all drugs, their actions and side effects]. Most people don't realize all the information in the *PDR* is provided by the drug companies—it's paid advertising.

"Naturally, they'd like to soft-pedal the negative side effects of a drug, and they do it in very sly ways. For instance, under amphetamines you'll find the warning: 'Do not prescribe to anyone with a history of drug addiction.' Well, that's like telling a car salesman not to sell cars to drunk drivers. How are they supposed to know who's had a history of addiction? The addicts aren't going to tell them."

The sheer volume of new information most doctors have to keep on top of makes it impossible for them to really understand much more than the few dozen drugs commonly used in their specialty, Dr. Levy says. Much of the questionable prescribing of Valium, adds Ms. Levin, has been done by internists and general practitioners, not psychiatrists, who would tend to be better informed about the uses and abuses of a drug best suited for psychiatric purposes. (In Barbara Gordon's case, however, it was a psychiatrist who got her into trouble.)

In the end, as in everything else concerning your health, *you* are the responsible party. If your physician is unaware of the long-term effects of a drug he or she prescribes for you, and you develop a dependence, it's *your* health that suffers, not your doctor's—and it's your fault for not having educated yourself about the chemical you were feeding your body. Good sources of information about drugs, according to Dr. Levy, include *The Essential Guide To Prescription Drugs,* by James W. Long, M.D. (Harper & Row, 1982), and Joe Graedon's "People's Pharmacy" books. The *PDR* is also available in many bookstores.

Good News Addendum

We're All Getting Younger

A decade ago, a reporter interviewing Gloria Steinem remarked with more sincerity than flattery that the feminist writer didn't look her age, which was 40.

"But this," responded Ms. Steinem, "is what 40 looks like."

Last year, Ms. Steinem, a founding editor of *Ms.* magazine, gave America a gander at what 50 looks like by posing in a bathtub for *People* magazine, a scene saved from being scandalous by a few well-placed suds.

The well-publicized photo might well become the pinup of a new generation of people who, like Ms. Steinem, appear to have slipped undetected behind the enemy lines of middle age.

This is what 50 looks like:

To celebrate her fiftieth birthday, actress Shirley MacLaine kicked up a shapely leg on the cover of *Time*—and picked up her first Oscar.

To mark his half century, California attorney David Pierce became a first-time father.

Head librarian Janet Glassman, who had never even jogged

until a few years ago, in her midfifties ran the 1984 Boston Marathon, where she set a new American record in her age group.

Gerald Carson had no sooner blown out the 50 candles on his cake than he quit his job as a New York advertising executive and embarked on a second career as a writer. He finished his tenth book over a year ago—at the age of 83.

And that is what 83 looks like.

Clearly, something revolutionary is happening to our concept of age. We are coming to think of the 28-year-old mayor, the 50-year-old first-time father and the 66-year-old weight lifter as commonplace. The old stereotypes are no longer serviceable. Who, for instance, would relegate a 60-year-old to a front-porch rocker if the 60-year-old in question were actor Paul Newman, who hits that milestone this year?

It's the kind of thing that would clear a carnival age-guesser's shelves of Kewpie dolls. We are becoming what noted gerontologist Bernice L. Neugarten, Ph.D., calls "an age-irrelevant society." Knowing an adult's age no longer gives us the rundown on the rest of his life. Age has been reduced to simple arithmetic.

"Age is a measure of the number of years you've been on the planet and not a measure of spirit," says Kaylan Pickford, the 54-year-old model whose seductive photos in her book, *Always a Woman* (Bantam, 1982), detonate the myth that middle age isn't sexy.

Not only is it sexy, there is increasing evidence that in our later years we become healthier, wealthier and wiser than anybody ever thought. Not only is there life after 40, the odds are that it's going to be better than life before.

What happened? The best answer comes from writer Ralph Schoenstein, who celebrated his fiftieth birthday by playing touch football with men just slightly older than some of his suits. When, at the end of the game, he wasn't carted off to a waiting ambulance, he said he knew he wasn't over the hill. "I knew," he said, "that the hill had been moved."

And no one is quite sure where it has been repositioned. People are not only thinking younger, they're staying younger longer, with all the health, life and vigor that implies.

In 1974, Louis Harris and the National Council on Aging

conducted a poll of men and women over 18, asking them, "At what age do you think the average individual becomes old?" The median age volunteered by the men was 63 and, by the women, 62. But seven years later, the median had climbed to 66 and 65 respectively. Some years earlier, a Duke University study asked 135 men and women over 60 how old they felt. More than half of the 60-to-69 age group said they felt young or middle-aged—and so did a quarter of those over 75.

Like statesman Bernard Baruch, most people apparently believed that old age is "15 years older than I am."

More significant, it may be true physiologically. Alvar Svanborg, M.D., a Swedish gerontologist, is in the midst of an ongoing study of 70-year-olds and has, so far, examined three successive groups five years apart. What he has found is that every successive group is physiologically younger than the previous group.

"Nobody knows why yet, but this is happening in all industrialized societies," says D. Lydia Bronte, Ph.D. Dr. Bronte is staff director of the Aging Society Project, a study sponsored by Carnegie Corporation of New York to gauge the impact of population aging on American society. So remarkable is the growth of this vital over-50 age group that the Aging Society Project's founder and chairman Alan Pifer believes that we have created a whole new life stage. Pifer has proposed a new name for the period from 50 to 75: He calls it the "Third Quarter of Life," a more appropriate replacement for the terms used now for people in this age group, like "senior citizen," which carry negative meanings.

One thing is certain: The presence of these active and vigorous older people will have a powerful influence on our national life. In the United States, the generation of over-45s, at 71 million strong, is nearly as large as the postwar Baby Boom generation, at 76 million the largest in history. In fact, according to the latest census figures, there are more people over 45 than there are children. Today, about three out of every ten Americans is what is known euphemistically as "mature." They and the Baby Boom generation, themselves just beginning to gray, are destined to spearhead a major social revolution, says Dr. Bronte. In time, we will stop worshipping youth and light a candle to maturity.

"The image ideal is already inching upward," she says. "I just got a catalog in the mail in which the models used to be very young. They still are, but this time there was one clearly in her fifties. It's starting to happen now. People are discovering the virtues of maturity."

One of those virtues is money—and it's been discovered by Madison Avenue. The New York advertising firm Jordan, Case & McGrath, Incorporated, recently published its study of the 55-plus market, calling it "the marketing opportunity of the 80s."

"We *are* the market," says Kaylan Pickford, whose silver hair and Caribbean-blue eyes have sold everything from wheat germ to furs since she began her modeling career at 45.

Indeed they are. According to a study by Compton Advertising of New York, the per capita income for households in which the head is between 50 and 64 is 39 percent higher than for households headed by younger wage earners. The latest census figures indicate full-time workers between the ages of 55 and 64 have incomes comparable to those of younger workers. But buying power is greater among the older group—by 15 percent—because of the smaller household size and fewer expenses that entails.

But what of the over-65s? The stereotype of those on fixed incomes is fraught with visions of cat-food suppers and unheated homesteads that wind up on the auction block for unpaid taxes. In this age group, the myths are strong and persistent. But the fact is, only 15 percent of the nation's elderly have incomes that fall below the poverty line. While that's more than the general population, the number of elderly poor has diminished more rapidly. One economic writer referred to this grossly misunderstood generation as "the wellderly," which can just as accurately describe their health as their financial status.

They are healthy. We are indeed living in a time of what University of Miami sociologist Aaron Lipman, Ph.D., calls "mass longevity." Multiply buying power by leisure years—an estimated 16 years after 65—and you get some concept of the real meaning of gray power.

"A man of 65 can expect to live to 79; 84 for women," says Richard Shepherd, executive director of the National Association of Mature People, a nonprofit group based in Oklahoma City. "And some people are opting to retire early at 55. That means there's a lot of living to be done."

Good health, brought on by quantum-leap advances in public health, is what many think is responsible. More people are growing older healthier. The 65-and-over population grew twice as fast as the rest of the population in the last 20 years, and four out of five of them are fit and mobile.

Though death and illness rates climb after 45, the majority of mature adults enjoy excellent health. For instance, though more than three-quarters of those over 65 report they are plagued by chronic illness, it may be no more serious than weakening eyesight or a touch of arthritis. "If you ask them how they feel, they'll say 'fine, considering my age,'" says Dr. Lipman.

According to a special report by the U.S. Census Bureau, eight in ten persons over 65 rate their health as "good" or "excellent." In fact, older people get fewer acute illnesses a year than younger people.

They are also increasingly drawn to America's fitness fever, even if the last time they tied on a pair of sneakers was 30 years ago in gym class. The National Senior Sports Association, which sponsors about 26 golf, tennis and bowling tournaments a year for older people, drew at least 2,200 entrants in its first year. The World Masters Track and Field Championships, open to competitors over 40, brought an unprecedented 2,000-plus older athletes to Gothenburg, Sweden, perhaps the largest single track meet ever held.

But older athletes aren't circumscribed by age brackets. When 56-year-old Janet Glassman, head librarian at Rodale Press, ran in last year's Boston Marathon, she didn't simply beat 18 women between the ages of 50 and 59. She placed 192 out of 582 women, most younger than she. "That means more to me than coming in first in my age group," she says. "The truth is, it always surprises me when I *can't* outrun the younger women. I always think I can."

Janet Glassman, like many of the other new-breed mid-lifers, follows what one author calls the "Satchel Paige principle." Baseball great Paige, who pitched in the major leagues until he was almost 50, once asked, "How old would you be if you didn't know how old you was?" More of these revolutionary mid-lifers are acting as if they don't know what age they are.

For that, says Dr. Bronte, they can thank a relaxation of some of the cultural expectations of aging.

Unlike their parents, the new midlifers don't regard any age as a signal to put away the things of their youth and bring out the lap robe and bifocals.

"My parents thought they were older when they were 50 than I think I am at this age," says David Pierce, holding his firstborn, Rio, on his lap.

This new attitude is allowing older people like David Pierce and Janet Glassman to literally age youthfully, to start families and run marathons when they are close to retirement age. And the attitude may be no more than recognition that the bogeyman of aging—physical and intellectual deterioration, senility and lack of sexual vigor—are not biological inevitabilities.

Twenty-five years of experiments with laboratory rats led California neuroanatomist Marian C. Diamond, Ph.D., to attack the notion that all brain nerve cells, which receive, transmit and store information, deteriorate with age. In fact, says the University of California professor, not only do cells in certain areas of the cerebral cortex not deteriorate, in an enriched environment they can actually grow. "We've found the potential of the aging brain is more optimistic than previously thought," says Dr. Diamond.

Another significant mental faculty, known as crystallized intelligence, has been shown to increase over the life span of a healthy adult. Crystallized intelligence is the ability to use stored information to solve problems, says researcher John Horn, Ph.D., a psychologist at the University of Denver. Older people have a greater ability than the young to tap into and use their storehouse of knowledge for problem solving. "There is some evidence that, at least in one sense, people become more and more intelligent throughout the years of adulthood," says Dr. Horn.

That is not to say there aren't some losses in intellectual abilities with age. There is a consistent decline is what is known as fluid intelligence. "This is the ability to confront novel conditions where the well-organized knowledge system is not applicable," says the psychologist.

But senility is rare (it's a disease occurring in only about 1 percent of the population) and intelligence as measured by standardized tests may actually increase. Several years ago, clinical psychologist Jon Kangas, Ph.D., did a follow-up study of 48 men and women whose intelligence had been tested in 1931, 1941, 1956 and 1969. He discovered that their IQs actually rose 20 points between childhood and middle age and he speculates that the climb can continue after middle age under the right circumstances.

Index

213

Rodale Press, Inc., publishes PREVENTION®, the better health magazine.
For information on how to order your subscription,
write to PREVENTION®, Emmaus, PA 18049.